Nutritional Epigenetics
Unsafe At Any Meal Study Guide

Nutritional Epigenetics
Unsafe At Any Meal Study Guide

by
Dr. Renee Joy Dufault

Copyright © 2023 by Renee Joy Dufault
All rights reserved. No part of this book may be reproduced, scanned,
or distributed in any printed or electronic form without permission.
First Edition: March 2023
Printed in the United States of America
ISBN: 9798885678742

For my children, grandchildren,
great grandchildren, and all the world's children.

Table of Contents

Acknowledgements, vii

Preface, viii

Purpose, ix

Introduction to Toxic Substances, Chapter 1, page 1

Genes and Your Health, Chapter 2, page 7

Pesticides and Adult-Onset Diseases, Chapter 3, page 13

Ingredients That Add Heavy Metals to Your Body, Chapter 4, page 19

Our Western Diet and Disease, Chapter 5, page 27

Spotlight on Autism and ADHD, Chapter 6, page 36

Food Labeling Practices, Chapter 7, page 45

Creating a Safe Food Environment at Home, Chapter 8, page 53

Answer Keys, page 59

About Dr. Dufault, page 65

References, page 69

Acknowledgements

This study guide would not be needed if it were not for the contaminated food supply in the United States (U.S.) and elsewhere. The continued use of food ingredients with allowable heavy metal residues remains a problem. In 2021, the U.S. Congress issued two separate reports on the levels of toxic heavy metals found in foods eaten by infants and children.

Since 2010, the non-profit Food Ingredient and Health Research Institute (FIHRI) has provided a virtual platform to support my research work and the dissemination of food ingredient safety information at no charge to the public. FIHRI has no paid staff, and all the work is done by volunteers. There are expenses associated with running a website, conducting research, and filing the required tax returns each year for a 501 c 3 non-profit organization. In addition, there are office expenses related to developing and giving presentations to the public or providing volunteer instruction for healthy diet workshops. If it were not for the small donations of my friends and family, FIHRI would not have been able to survive as an entity all these years. I am so grateful to my family members and friends.

I would also like to thank the following FIHRI supporters for their generous track record of tangible giving in the form of time, resources, or funding: Dr. Raquel Crider, Dr. Zara Berg, Dr. Steven Gilbert, Fort Peck Community College, the Volcano Friends Feeding Friends, Men of Pa'a, Hawai'i Community Foundation, Jillian Hishaw of F.A.R.M.S., Dr. Skip Kingston, Dr. Mesay Mulugeta Wolle, Dr. Walter Lukiw, Katsi Cook, Dr. David Carpenter, Dr. Katherine Adler, Amanda Hitt of the Government Accountability Project Food Integrity Campaign, and last but not least, Dr. Roseanne Schnoll.

Preface

When I originally published *Unsafe at Any Meal: What the FDA Does Not Want You to Know About the Foods You Eat* in 2017, it never occurred to me that the book would be used by colleges as a textbook for nutritional epigenetics and health education courses. My strategy for getting the word out about the contaminants in the food supply was to develop a free online Healthy Diet tutorial to go with the book. The free tutorial was published at the Food Ingredient and Health Research Institute website in 2017. The Healthy Diet tutorial was available online for many years. When it became apparent the tutorial was not being used by the public, I decided to write this study guide to go with the book instead. If colleges were going to use the book as a textbook, then students could surely benefit from having a study guide that not only went with the textbook but also included content from FIHRI's successful online Healthy Diet tutorials.

This study guide incorporates most of the content of the online healthy diet tutorials developed and used by FIHRI as interventions in three different clinical trials to help participants successfully switch to a healthier eating pattern. Native American college students who participated in the Fort Peck Community College trials switched to a healthier eating pattern, lost weight, reduced BMI, and lowered their blood inorganic mercury and glucose levels. The clinical trial involving parents of children with autism and/or ADHD was also successful with measured improvements in family diets.

As you read the *Unsafe at Any Meal* textbook, you will use this study guide to improve your understanding of the components in the western diet that impact the way your genes behave. Your diet will introduce factors that interact with your genes to either protect your health or make you more susceptible to disease. The study of these dietary factors that influence gene behavior is known as nutritional epigenetics. Topics under study will include gene-environment interactions, changes in dietary consumption patterns over time, allowable toxic substance levels in food ingredients, regulatory role of the U.S. Food and Drug Administration (FDA), conventional vs organic foods, micronutrients, and components of a healthy diet.

You will learn how to identify environmental and dietary factors that impact gene regulation leading to improvements in health or the development of disease. You will examine western dietary pattern over the last forty years and determine changes in the overall consumption of specific foods and food ingredients. You will survey kitchen cupboards, refrigerator, and freezer to identify food or food ingredients containing toxic substances that may impact gene function. You will recognize resources for improving family diet and health. You will essentially create a healthy food environment at your home.

With this study guide and the book *Unsafe at Any Meal: What the FDA Does Not Want You to Know About the Foods You Eat It*, you will embark on a life changing self-guided tour of the western food supply.

Purpose

The purpose of this study guide is to help you master the subject of nutritional epigenetics that is presented at the introductory level in the textbook *Unsafe at Any Meal: What the FDA Does Not Want You to Know About the Foods You Eat* (see book cover below). The textbook is available for purchase in bookstores or online via amazon.com. The textbook and study guide together may serve as ready to use curriculum in a college course, community health education setting, book study group, or as part of a healthy diet intervention.

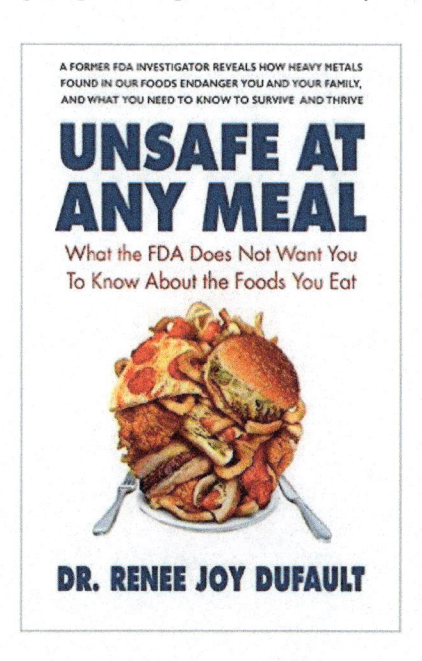

In this study guide, modules of instruction include learning objectives, activities, and discussion questions for each chapter in the textbook. Each module of instruction includes a reading guide to enhance comprehension and learning. As a strategy for success, I highly recommend the reader complete the reading guides provided for each chapter **before** moving on to the activities. Discussion questions are designed to enhance small group learning. The study guide is developed using differentiated instructional techniques. Through differentiated instruction, readers will be able to master the concepts and teach others about the influence of dietary factors on gene behavior.

Module 1

Introduction to Toxic Substances

During this module of instruction, you will learn how a substance becomes toxic or unsafe. Many substances do not become harmful until a threshold of exposure is reached, and your body reacts. Every human being is genetically different. Infants, children, and the elderly are sensitive populations in which toxic substance exposures can cause more harm. Parents need to take a precautionary approach in feeding their children. An exposure to a substance may be safe for one person but toxic to another.

LEARNING OBJECTIVES

1. Describe what makes a substance toxic.

2. Recognize the current risk assessment process is not reliable.

3. Describe the dangers of over-fluoridation.

4. Explain how the bioaccumulation of heavy metals may occur in your body.

5. Explain why toxic substances are dangerous to health.

ACTIVITIES

1. As you read Chapter 1 of your textbook, complete the Chapter 1 Reading Guide provided in this study guide on pages 3-6.

2. Visit the Centers for Disease Control (CDC) website. Determine the allowable fluoride levels in your drinking water supply. **Key words** for Google search are "**MWF and CDC and My Water's Fluoride**." NOTE: If you do not live in the U.S., find out if there is fluoride in your water supply.

https://nccd.cdc.gov/doh_mwf/default/default.aspx

Dr. Renee Joy Dufault

3. Survey your kitchen cupboard to identify what kind of flour you use. Read the ingredient label. Is the flour bleached? _____

4. Find the manufacturing specifications for the chlorine used to bleach flour at the United Nations FAO website. **Key words** for enabling search on Google are "**FAO and chlorine monograph**." Download PDF file titled **Chlorine**. Scroll down second page to find the allowable mercury and lead levels.

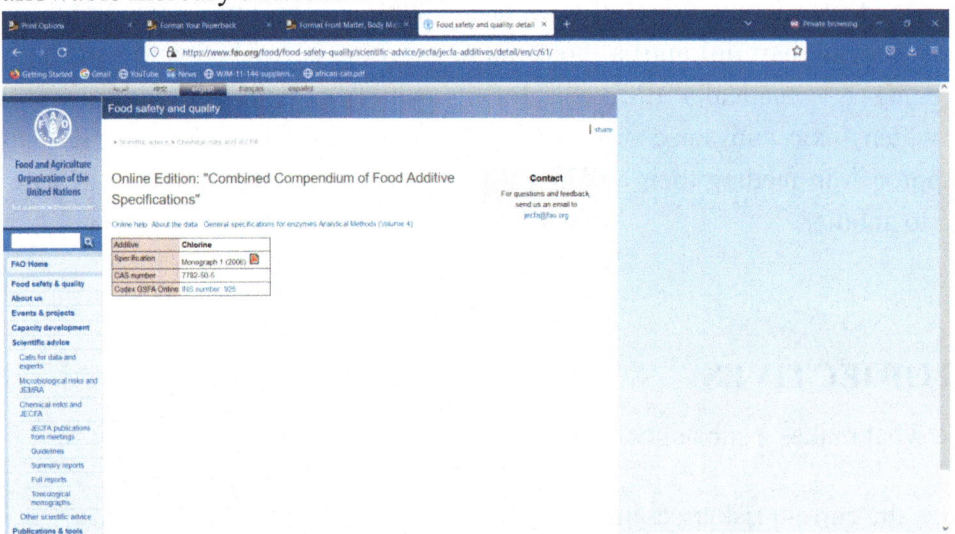

https://www.fao.org/food/food-safety-quality/scientific-advice/jecfa/jecfa-additives/detail/en/c/61/

STUDY GROUP DISCUSSION QUESTIONS

- What is the danger of fluoride in drinking water? Is any amount of exposure safe? Can fluoride bioaccumulate?

  _____

- How can you be exposed to inorganic mercury or lead from the food you eat? Give examples of food products that may contain trace amounts of inorganic mercury or lead based on what you learned about bleached flour.

  _____

- Eating refined white flour foods (e.g., bread, bagels, cookies, pastries) has been shown to significantly increase blood glucose (sugar) levels in people with Type 1 and Type 2 diabetes. Do you think the mercury in the bleached flour might be a risk factor for developing Type-2 diabetes?

  _____

Reading Guide for Chapter 1, Module 1

Directions: Please answer the following questions as you are reading Chapter 1 of your textbook.

What makes a substance toxic?

1. When caffeine is **added** to food, it must be listed on the list of ingredients. True or False

2. There is a limit on the amount of caffeine that can be added to a food. The limit is _____

3. Caffeine can cause death when eaten in amounts lower than the allowable levels by certain people such as those with _____ or _____ disease.

4. FDA has set a safe limit of exposure to caffeine for children and teens. True or False

5. Caffeine is now sometimes added to which of the following products:
    a. Jellybeans
    b. Marshmallows
    c. Sunflower seeds
    d. All the above

6. The toxicity of a substance cannot be defined by an allowable exposure limit. True or False

Risk Assessment and Safe Substances

7. The risk assessment process is the process used to find out if a substance is safe or not. True or False

8. If there are no studies available or literature on the safety of a substance, then it is deemed "safe." True or False

9. When can water become toxic or unsafe to drink? Give two examples.
   _____
   _____

Upper Limits

10. In the case of food toxicants, a common guideline for allowable exposure is the _____ limit.

11. The upper limit of a substance is the amount that can be eaten with no harmful effect over a 24-hour period. True or False

12. The problem with the current risk assessment system is that is does not consider the toxic effects that may occur over time such as continuous exposure to tiny amounts of lead in a contaminated drinking water system.   True or False

13. Define "bioaccumulation."
_____
_____

14. As we learn more about the harmful effects of bioaccumulation, the upper limits of exposure change for substances of concern. Allowable levels or upper limits of fluoride in drinking water have _____ (increased or decreased).

15. Scientists have determined there is no safe level of exposure for lead. Is the same true for fluoride? Do you think there is a safe level of exposure for fluoride?
_____
_____

COMPLETE Activity 2 for Module One. There is a CDC link that takes you to a website that tracks fluoride levels in drinking water supplies.

16. What did you find out about the fluoride level in your drinking water supply?
_____
_____

Arsenic

17. Arsenic is a problem contaminant in rice. It is important to know where the rice you buy is grown.   True or False

Cadmium

18. It is a clever idea for women to smoke cigarettes during pregnancy.   True or False

19. Cadmium can impact _____ and Vitamin D metabolism.

Lead

20. There is no safe level of exposure to lead. What does the bioaccumulation of lead to the elderly population?
_____
_____

Mercury

COMPLETE Activity 3 for Module One. Survey your kitchen cupboard to determine what type of flour you use. Is your flour bleached? Describe your flour product here _____

21. Chemicals are used to make processed foods. Chlorine or chlor-alkali chemicals (caustic soda or sodium hydroxide, hydrogen chloride) may be used to
   a. regulate the food product's acid levels
   b. regulate the food product's pH level to prevent it from spoiling
   c. all the above

22. GRAS is an acronym used by the FDA that means "generally _____ as _____."

23. Chlorine or chlor-alkali products made using mercury have inorganic mercury residues in them. True   or   False

24. Organic mercury is different than the inorganic mercury because it has a carbon molecule attached to it. Which kind of mercury can be found in fish tissue?
   _____

Why are toxic substances dangerous?

25. Arsenic, cadmium, lead and mercury are heavy metals that can bioaccumulate in your body over time leading to the development of western diseases such as (list three diseases of greatest concern to you)
   _____
   _____
   _____

26. Exposures to toxic metals interferes with _____ function or behavior.

Tainting the food supply

27. Which three (3) chemicals will you NOT find on a food ingredient label?
   _____, _____, and _____.

Chlorine

COMPLETE Activity 4 for Module One. Did you find the PDF file on the FAO website that provides the specification for the allowable mercury in chlorine used to bleach flour? Describe your finding here. _____

28. Bleached flour is white due to the use of chlorine in its processing. True   or   False

29. The chlorine used to bleach flour has an allowable mercury level of _____.

Hydrogen chloride

30. Hydrogen chloride can be made with the mercury cell process or some other manufacturing process. True   or   False

Sodium hydroxide (also known as caustic soda)

31. Sodium hydroxide is used in making vegetable oils. In 2012, the average American ate _____ pounds of vegetable oil.

Measuring toxic load

32. Biomarkers are substances in your body that can be collected to measure how much heavy metal you have in your body. Give four examples of biomarker substances (blood is one). _____, _____, _____, and _____.

33. Based on your understanding of Chapter 1, a substance becomes toxic when _____ _____

Reflect on what you found most surprising about what you learned during Module 1.
_____
_____
_____

Healthy diet tip for today! Buy unbleached **organic flour and keep it in your refrigerator**. It lasts forever and is so much healthier!! See text box below to learn more!!

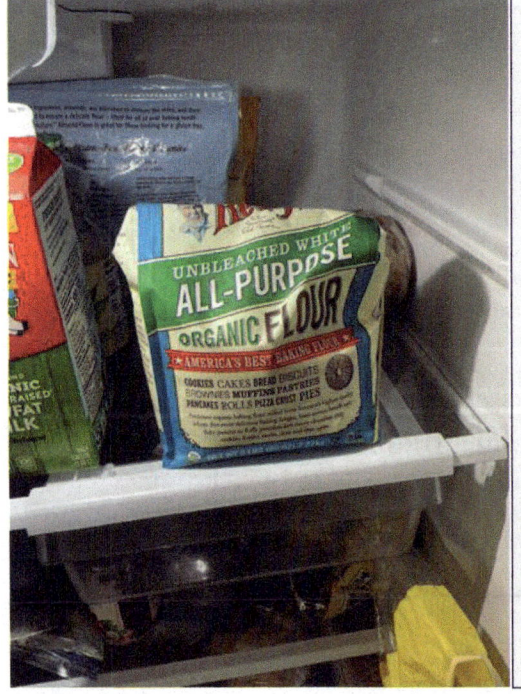

Organic vs Conventionally Grown Wheat Flour

Organic flour must be stored in the refrigerator, or it will mold. This type of flour is made from wheat stored in *refrigerated* silos where pesticides are NOT applied to prevent insects from laying their eggs. Insect egg hatching is controlled via temperature. Bleach is, by definition, a pesticide because it kills mold. Since organic flour cannot contain pesticides, it is unbleached. By law, the organic wheat can only be stored in the refrigerated silos for up to one year.

Conventionally grown wheat can be stored in silos for up to five years and pesticides (e.g., malathion and other organophosphate pesticides) are applied to it as often as needed to prevent insects and eggs from hatching.

Module 2

Genes and Your Health

During this module of instruction, you will learn how your diet and environment influences the way your genes behave or express themselves. The study of these "gene-environment interactions" is called *epigenetics*. Understanding the dietary factors that influence gene expression is key to maintaining good health and preventing disease.

LEARNING OBJECTIVES

1. Describe the importance of, and mechanisms for, building methylation capacity.

2. Recognize the importance of dietary calcium in carrying out the functions of the PON1 and BDNF genes.

3. Recognize the role of dietary zinc in carrying out the function of the MT gene.

4. Describe the gene environment interactions associated with autism and Alzheimer's disease.

5. Describe the role of dietary calcium in the elimination of lead from the body and the prevention of ADHD.

ACTIVITIES

1. As you read Chapter 2 of your textbook complete the Chapter 2 Reading Guide provided on pages 10-12 of this study guide. Be sure to complete your reading guide **before** watching the video.

2. View the video titled "Ghost in Your Genes" that is uploaded on dailymotion.com (with ads) for free. You can also view this awesome video on PBS with a subscription.

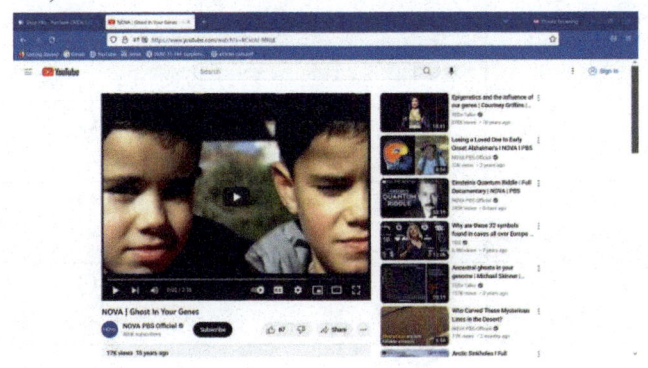

Link to PBS here: https://www.youtube.com/watch?v=KCvcnJ-MRqE

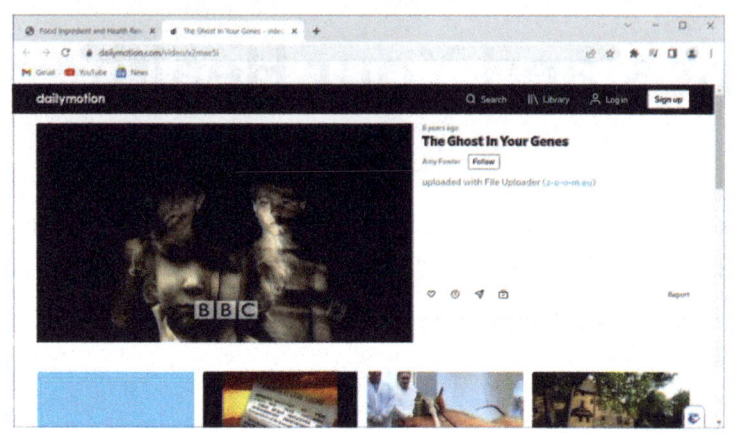

Link to dailymotion.com upload: https://www.dailymotion.com/video/x2mwr5i

What was the takeaway lesson for you when you finished watching the Ghost in Your Genes video?

_____
_____
_____

3. Use an Internet search engine (e.g., Google, Yahoo) to find foods rich in zinc and rich in calcium. List foods in the table below and survey your kitchen for their presence:

Foods rich in zinc	Present? (circle)	Foods rich in calcium	Present? (circle)
	YES/NO		YES/NO
	YES/NO		YES/NO
	YES/NO		YES/NO
	YES/NO		YES/NO
	YES/NO		YES/NO
	YES/NO		YES/NO
	YES/NO		YES/NO
	YES/NO		YES/NO

STUDY GROUP DISCUSSION QUESTIONS

- What is methylation and why is it important in disease prevention?
  _____
  _____

- Describe two genes involved in autism and Alzheimer's disease and the factors that may influence their activity or the way they function.
  _____
  _____
  _____

- Based on your Internet findings and kitchen survey, what measures can you take to improve your dietary environment?
  _____
  _____
  _____

Healthy diet tip for today! A one cup (8-ounce) serving of **moringa leaves** contains nearly four times the amount of calcium of an 8-ounce cup of milk. Moringa is also rich in iron, zinc, Vitamin A, protein, potassium, and Vitamin C. For this reason, it is used throughout the world to cure malnutrition in children under the age of three years.

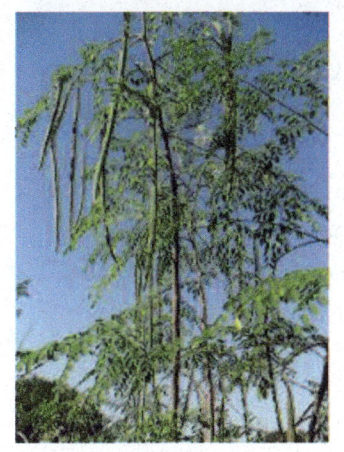

Asian and African cultures have long known about the nutritional benefits of eating Moringa. The Moringa tree is called the "miracle tree" because parts of it are harvested and used as medicines throughout the world to cure Type-1 and Type-2 diabetes, cancer, and dementia.[1]

The Moringa tree is easy to grow in hot or warm tropical climates (e.g., dry side of tropical Hawaiian Islands, Arizona, California). The pods can be cut up and cooked in the same way you would cook string beans. The pods also provide seeds for growing more Moringa trees.

Moringa leaves can be eaten raw in a smoothie, cooked in a soup, or dried in the oven for later use as a powder.

Moringa Smoothie Recipe Ingredients: 2 cups organic milk (any kind), ½ cup fresh moringa leaves or 1 tbsp. moringa powder, 1 banana (can be fresh or frozen).

Directions: Add milk, fresh moringa leaves (or powder) and frozen banana to a blender. Blend until creamy. Makes one serving.

Dr. Renee Joy Dufault

Reading Guide for Chapter 2, Module 2

Directions: Please answer the following questions as you are reading Chapter 2 of your textbook.

Genes and Your Health

1. Your genes do not run on gasoline; they run on the air you breathe, the water you drink and the food you eat.   True   or   False

2. What you eat and drink provides chemical elements (e.g., zinc, calcium, magnesium, arsenic, mercury, lead, etc....) that determine how your genes behave. True   or   False

What do genes do?

3. Genes provide the instructions for your cells, so they know what to do. Give an example of a type of cell and an instruction it might have been given to do a certain job. (Hint: Think of the different organs in your body and what they do for you).
   _____

4. Genes turn on or off telling cells what to do. A cell can become cancerous or stay healthy and carry out its job. One process that turns your genes on or off is _____.

5. Where are genes located? _____

Cell Differentiation

6. _____ is when a cell decides what kind of cell it will be and what it will do.

7. A liver cell will function in response to its environment. With over-consumption of the drug "alcohol," liver cells will become overworked in trying to breakdown the alcohol. They will become sick. The following are liver diseases that can develop from drinking too much alcohol:
   a. fatty liver
   b. hepatitis
   c. cirrhosis
   d. all the above

8. The study of how genes (inside your cells) respond to the environment in your body is _____.

9. A parent can pass on the way their genes work to their children.   True   or   False

Methylation

10. A methyl group is made up of one carbon atom and two hydrogen atoms. True   or   False

11. What happens if a methyl group is added to a gene?
    a. The gene may turn off
    b. The gene may turn on
    c. The gene may start to produce a protein
    d. The gene may stop producing a protein
    e. All the above

12. Your body can have too many methyl groups or not enough.   True   or   False

13. Proteins are important! For example, in a child's body, proteins are used to help the child speak. In an adult, proteins help maintain memory.   True   or   False

14. The _____ you eat determines how many methyl groups your body will have to work with.

15. Certain nutrients donate methyl groups. Give three examples. _____, _____, and _____.

16. What are some diseases that occur when a body does not have enough methyl groups or if it is hypomethylated? List three of greatest concern to you. _____, _____, and _____.

17. Look at Table 5.3 on page 90. Of the methyl donating foods listed, which do you eat a lot of?
_____

COMPLETE Activity 2 for Module 2. The video "Ghost in Your Genes" is a great introduction to how genes can switch off and on via methylation patterns.

The Importance of Genes

18. What kind of genes cause cancer? _____

19. Oncogenes will turn on with exposure to certain things or agents, including
    a. exposure to some viruses
    b. exposure to UV rays from the sun
    c. exposure to certain pesticides
    d. all the above

20. What kind of gene will stop a tumor from growing? _____

21. In a healthy body, oncogenes are kept in check by _____ and _____.

22. Vitamin D plays a role in silencing the cancer genes.   True   or   False

23. In each cell of the human body, there are about 21,000 genes. We don't know much about most of them. The good news is we do know ALOT about a few of them. In Chapter 2, I talk about three of them. Below is a chart: Fill it out and show me what you know.

Short name (acronym)	Long name (protein)	Your body uses this protein to _____.
MT		
		attach memories to brain cells.
	Paraoxonase-1	

24. BDNF is calcium dependent. Children with autism have lower BDNF levels. What nutrient are they not getting enough of? _____ Google and give three examples of foods rich in this nutrient. _____, _____, and _____.

25. Alzheimer's and dementia are both found in people that do not have enough paraoxonase in their bodies to break down organophosphate pesticide residues found in conventional foods. What nutrient is PON1 dependent on? _____

26. What organ in your body makes paraoxonase enzyme?
    a. liver
    b. heart
    c. lungs

27. PON1 gene activity and paraoxonase levels are lower in
    a. boys compared to girls
    b. elderly people
    c. people with Alzheimer's or dementia
    d. children with autism and ADHD
    e. all the above

28. MT genes provide your cells with the instructions to make the protein metallothionein. What nutrient is MT dependent on? _____

29. Zinc deficiency is common in _____ disease, autism and _____.

30. Metal transporter proteins like the MT help your body get rid of toxic heavy metals. What happens if your diet does not include enough zinc rich foods?
_____

31. After the PON1 gene makes the paraoxonase enzyme in your liver cell, where does the paraoxonase end up? Hint: It joins up with a healthy cholesterol. This protein (good cholesterol) is something your doctor will test for. What is it? _____

Module 3

Pesticides and Adult-Onset Diseases

During this module of instruction, you will learn how pesticide exposures occur and their role in creating conditions for the development of the more common neurological and/or metabolic disorders such as autism, Alzheimer's, and ADHD.

LEARNING OBJECTIVES

1. Recognize the agricultural commodities most likely to contain organophosphate pesticide residues.

2. Describe how chlorine is used as a pesticide in agricultural and food manufacturing processes.

3. Explain how co-exposures can impact health and the environment.

4. Become familiar with the role of certain pesticides in creating the problem of antibiotic resistant organisms or super bacteria.

5. Explain how you can eliminate or reduce your exposure to pesticides.

ACTIVITIES

1. As you read Chapter 3 of your textbook, complete the Chapter 3 Reading Guide provided in this study guide on pages 15-17.

2. Review the references for Chapter 3 of your textbook listed between pages 180 and 184. Choose three references of interest to you and look them up on the internet. What are your thoughts on each? Does the reference(s) support the text you read?

   _____
   _____
   _____

3. Survey your kitchen cupboards and refrigerator and make a list of all the foods likely to contain pesticide residues (e.g., products made from corn or wheat, vegetables, fruits, other?).

   _____

Dr. Renee Joy Dufault

_____
_____

STUDY GROUP DISCUSSION QUESTIONS

- What evidence is there to suggest pesticide exposure is linked to the development of neurological disease? Provide two references.
_____
_____

- What are examples of co-exposures and how might they impact health or development?
_____
_____

- Based on your kitchen survey findings, share what you can do to reduce your exposure to pesticides.
_____
_____
_____

Healthy diet tip for today! Buy triple rinsed organic greens to reduce your pesticide exposure! If you are busy working fulltime and must rely on some convenience foods to get you through your work week, consider buying triple rinsed organic greens. This pre-packaged vegetable will help you meet your healthy diet goals. Go for a mix that includes spinach. Spinach is rich in both calcium and methyl group donating nutrients. You can't go wrong with triple rinsed greens that make it easy to prepare and eat a nutritious salad every day.

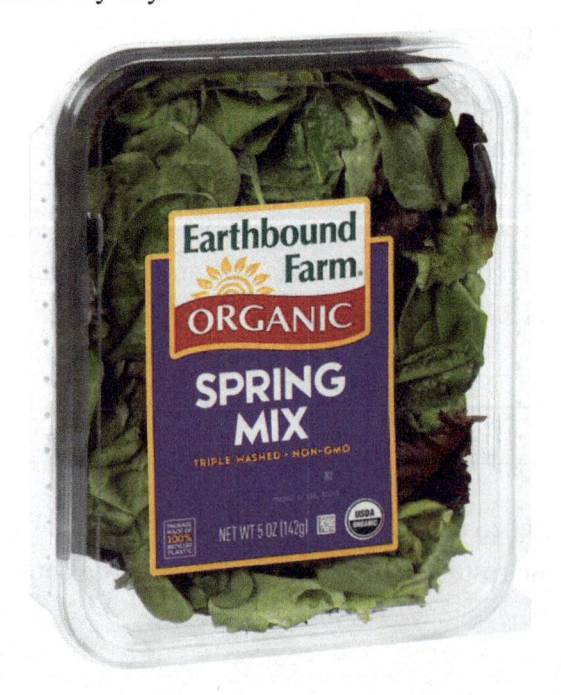

Reading Guide for Chapter 3, Module 3

Directions: Please answer the following questions as you are reading Chapter 3.

Pesticides and an Inside Look at Chlorine

1. Pesticides serve a variety of purposes, and each contains an ingredient that is toxic to the target organism. True or False

2. Chlorine is regulated by the _____ in the United States and may be used as a _____ to kill bacteria or a _____ to kill mold.

3. Organic farmers use pesticides. True or False

4. Organic crops in the U. S. are not allowed to contain pesticide residues. True or False

5. "Triple rinsed" lettuce is lettuce that has been rinsed three times with potable drinking water; the final rinse may not contain more than the allowable level of _____ in drinking water.

6. Chlorine (or bleach) is NOT a factor in the development of "super bacteria" that are much harder to kill with antibiotics. True or False

7. The following actions can be taken to reduce your risk of being infected by a "super bacteria:"
    a. Dechlorinate your tap or drinking water using a carbon filter (Brita).
    b. Avoid eating bleached flour and products made from bleached flour.
    c. Rinse vegetables and fruits well with dechlorinated drinking water.
    d. All the above

How Pesticide Exposure Happens

8. Bleached flour may contain inorganic mercury residues. True or False

9. If it is NOT organic, wheat flour can contain which of the following substances that may cause harm to the body over time:
    a. malathion pesticide residues
    b. chlorpyrifos pesticide residues
    c. inorganic mercury residues (if it is bleached)
    d. all the above

10. Can unbleached flour still contain pesticide residues even though it's not bleached?
    _____

Dr. Renee Joy Dufault

Pesticide Data Problem

11. The PDP is the USDA program that tracks pesticide residues in ag products. True or False

12. In 2012, the average American ate 95.1 pounds of wheat each year according to the United States Department of Agriculture (USDA). True or False

13. Fill in the blanks to explain the problems with the Pesticide Data Program.
    a. The PDP mostly focuses its pesticide residue testing efforts on fruits and _____. Grain crops are not tested every year even though people eat a lot of grains. The grain that is most often **eaten** is _____. Here in the United States many meals and snacks ("grain end products") are made with this grain (e.g., donuts, crackers, pizza crust, toast, hamburger buns, hotdog buns, noodles, cereal).

14. Reflect on your daily diet. Do you eat more rice or wheat end products in a typical week? Examples of end products include noodles, cereals, crackers, breads.
    _____
    _____

Pesticide Co-Exposure and Public Health

15. A co-exposure is when you are exposed to more than one potentially harmful substance at one time. Think about how a co-exposure to a pesticide and heavy metal may occur. For example, eating a bowl of highly processed cereal (e.g. Froot Loops) may easily lead to co-exposures. Look at the ingredients label for a cereal you may have in your cupboard or see page 49 of your textbook. List ingredients in this cereal that can lead to co-exposures (e.g., heavy metal, pesticides).
    _____
    _____
    _____

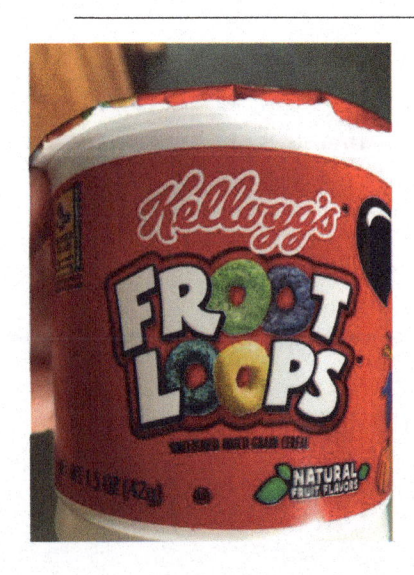

16. Your textbook *Unsafe at Any Meal: What the FDA Does Not Want You to Know About the Foods You Eat* was published in 2017. There have been some changes in the study of co-exposures and gene-environment interactions. Is there now a model that can be used to determine how co-exposures to heavy metals impact child health over time? (**HINT**: Find and read Dr. Dufault's 2023 publication in the World Journal of Clinical Pediatrics.) Please answer the question in the space provided below:

___

Pesticides and Neurological Disease

17. Scientists have linked exposures to individual pesticides to the development of Alzheimer's disease and Parkinson's disease. True or False

18. Which of the following heavy metal exposures also play a role in the development of Alzheimer's disease:

    a. lead
    b. arsenic
    c. carbon
    d. both a and b

19. Diet does NOT play a role in the development of Alzheimer's disease. True or False

Pesticides and Metabolic Disease (Type-2 Diabetes)

20. Patients with Type-2 diabetes have a higher risk of cancer because extra or excess glucose (sugar) in the blood feeds cancer cells. True or False

21. You can do at least three things to reduce your risk of developing Type-2 diabetes and cancer. List them here.
    _____
    _____

22. How can you keep organic flour from becoming moldy or infested with bug?
    _____
    _____

23. Do you think switching to an organic diet may improve your family's health? Explain.
    _____
    _____

Brainstorming Notes

Use this space to write down your thoughts and ideas on what you can do with the information you are learning. As you become more knowledgeable about the role unhealthy diet plays in the development of disease, how can you share this new information with others?

Module 4

Ingredients That Add Heavy Metals to Your Body

During this module of instruction, you will identify the most common food ingredients that contain allowable heavy metal residues. Scientists have determined that the concentration of heavy metals in food stuffs eaten by humans correlate directly with the heavy metals found in their bloodstream. We now know such exposures increase your risk of developing certain diseases such as Type-2 diabetes. Recent clinical trial data gathered throughout the world confirms children with autism always have higher levels of mercury and lead in their blood and children with ADHD always have higher levels of lead in their blood compared to healthy children without these disorders.

LEARNING OBJECTIVES

1. Recognize the food ingredients that contain allowable heavy metals (e.g., lead, inorganic mercury, cadmium, arsenic).

2. Describe how heavy metals may be introduced to food ingredients (e.g. vegetable oils, corn sweeteners, food colors.)

3. Explain how exposures to certain heavy metals may lead to changes in zinc status.

4. Become familiar with recipes for preparing zinc rich meals.

5. Review U.S. Congressional reports on heavy metals in the baby food supply.

ACTIVITIES

1. As you read Chapter 4 of your textbook, complete the Chapter 4 Reading Guide provided in this study guide on pages 23-26.

2. Using the list of foods high in zinc that you created during Module 2 (on page 8 of this workbook), do a keyword search on the internet to find a recipe that incorporates three or more foods on your high zinc food list. Shop for the ingredients, follow the recipe and prepare and eat the meal.

3. Visit Dr. Dufault's website http://www.reneedufault.com/ and scroll down to the bottom of the page to review at least one of the two reports published in 2021 by the U.S. Congress. Each report can be accessed by clicking on the associated picture →

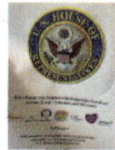

   What did you learn from reading one of these reports?
   _____
   _____
   _____

4. Using the tables provided in Chapter 4 of your textbook, survey your kitchen cupboards and refrigerator to find and list all the food products that may contain ingredients with at least one heavy metal impurity (use the chart on the next page to record your results). You will need to read the ingredient labels. For example, the food ingredient label below contains two ingredients with allowable or known heavy metal residues:

   INGREDIENTS: Premium brewed green tea, high fructose corn syrup, honey, citric acid, natural flavors, ginseng extract, vitamin C.

   Below is a label for Froot Loops:

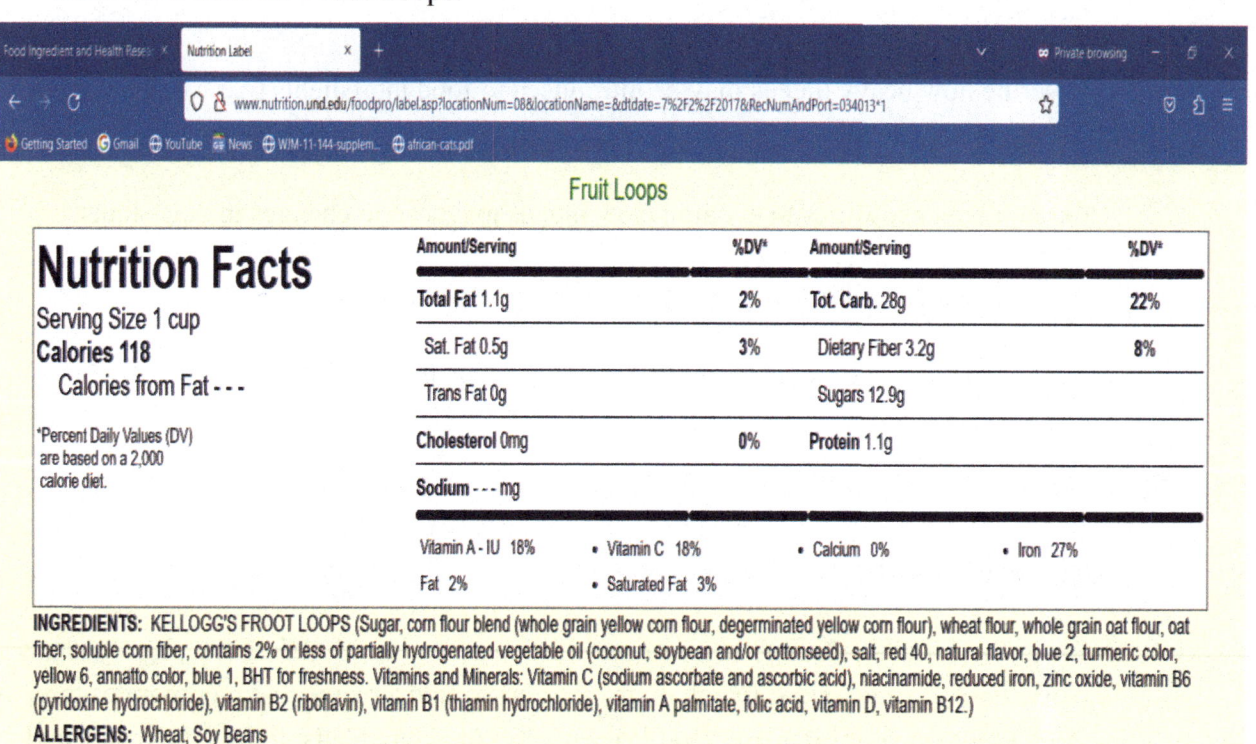

   Fruit Loops

   Nutrition Facts
   Serving Size 1 cup
   Calories 118
   Calories from Fat - - -

   *Percent Daily Values (DV) are based on a 2,000 calorie diet.

Amount/Serving	%DV*	Amount/Serving	%DV*
Total Fat 1.1g	2%	Tot. Carb. 28g	22%
Sat. Fat 0.5g	3%	Dietary Fiber 3.2g	8%
Trans Fat 0g		Sugars 12.9g	
Cholesterol 0mg	0%	Protein 1.1g	
Sodium - - - mg			

   Vitamin A - IU 18% • Vitamin C 18% • Calcium 0% • Iron 27%
   Fat 2% • Saturated Fat 3%

   INGREDIENTS: KELLOGG'S FROOT LOOPS (Sugar, corn flour blend (whole grain yellow corn flour, degerminated yellow corn flour), wheat flour, whole grain oat flour, oat fiber, soluble corn fiber, contains 2% or less of partially hydrogenated vegetable oil (coconut, soybean and/or cottonseed), salt, red 40, natural flavor, blue 2, turmeric color, yellow 6, annatto color, blue 1, BHT for freshness. Vitamins and Minerals: Vitamin C (sodium ascorbate and ascorbic acid), niacinamide, reduced iron, zinc oxide, vitamin B6 (pyridoxine hydrochloride), vitamin B2 (riboflavin), vitamin B1 (thiamin hydrochloride), vitamin A palmitate, folic acid, vitamin D, vitamin B12.)
   ALLERGENS: Wheat, Soy Beans

FOODS IN MY CUPBOARD WITH HEAVY METAL RESIDUES

Name of product	Food ingredient(s) with allowable or reported heavy metal residues
e.g., Fruit Loops	Vegetable (soybean) oil, red 40, blue 2, yellow 6, annatto, blue 1

STUDY GROUP DISCUSSION QUESTIONS

- What evidence is there to suggest that consumption of highly processed food contributes to your heavy metal exposure? Provide a reference to support your response.

_____
_____

- How does heavy metal exposure impact MT gene function and your body's zinc status? From your survey findings which food ingredients can you eliminate you're your diet to improve your zinc status?

_____
_____

- Share with a friend or family member the recipe you followed to prepare your zinc rich meal. Which ingredients were high in zinc? How did the meal turn out?

_____
_____
_____
_____

Need to find a healthy high zinc recipe? Try this one - Oat Bran Banana Bread

Ingredients: 2 eggs, ½ cup maple syrup, ½ cup organic plain (or honey flavored) Greek yogurt, 2-3 mashed bananas, 1 ¼ cup organic flour, 1 cup organic oat bran, 1 tsp. baking soda, ½ tsp salt, 1 tsp. cinnamon, 1 cup walnuts (or pecans)

Instructions: Preheat oven to 350 degrees, grease a loaf pan. In a large bowl or blender, mix eggs, maple syrup, yogurt, and banana. In a separate bowl, mix flour, oat bran, baking soda, salt and cinnamon. Add blended wet ingredients to flour mixture. Stir well. Blend in nuts. Pour into greased loaf pan and place in oven. Bake for 1 hour or until a knife can be inserted and pulled out clean.

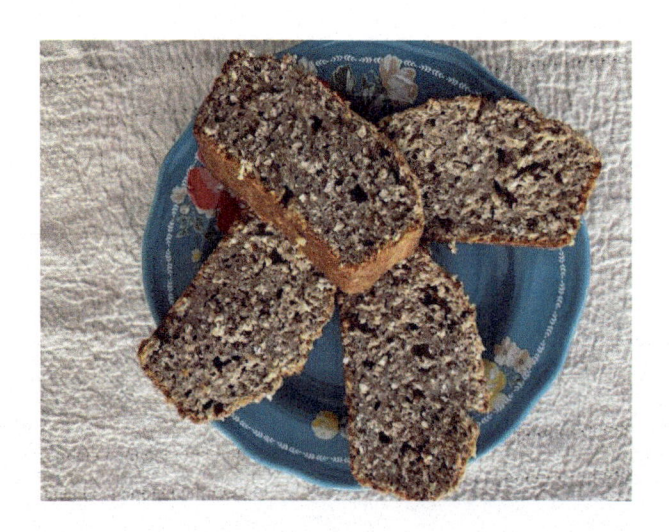

Reading Guide for Chapter 4, Module 4

Directions: Please answer the following questions as you are reading Chapter 4 of your textbook.

Ingredients That Add Heavy Metals to Your Body

1. The most common heavy metals found as residues in the food supply include which of the following:
   a. lead
   b. inorganic mercury
   c. cadmium
   d. arsenic
   e. all the above

2. The levels of heavy metals in foods eaten by adults and children match the heavy metal levels found in their blood. True or False

3. Explain why increasing heavy metal levels in blood can become a problem as you age.
   _____
   _____

Vegetable Oils

4. The average American consumes 16 pounds of vegetable oil each year. True or False

5. What is FEDIOL and what report did they publish?
   _____
   _____

6. Inorganic mercury can get into refined vegetable oils when a mercury cell chlor-alkali chemical is used in the manufacturing process to improve the taste of the oils. True or False

7. How has the amount of cooking oil eaten by Americans changed since 1970 compared to 2010 (Hint: see Table 4.2 to see pounds per person (capita) per year)?
   _____
   _____

8. In 2010 the average American ate 49.4 pounds of combined vegetable oil and fats. True or False

9. Vegetable oils are found in many products; examples of such products include
   a. salad dressings
   b. cookies
   c. mayonnaise
   d. all the above

23

10. Eating too much vegetable oil promotes the development of _____ disease and _____.

Corn Sweeteners

11. What compound is deliberately added to corn starch to prevent the production of enzymes by bacteria? _____

12. The corn sweetener manufacturing process involves the use of a mercury compound called *mercuric chloride*. True or False

13. Which of the following are corn sweeteners that may contain mercury residue?

    a. corn syrup
    b. dextrose
    c. high fructose corn syrup
    d. maltodextrin
    e. modified corn starch
    f. all the above

Inorganic Mercury Exposure from Eating Corn Sweeteners

14. What evidence shows that eating a lot of food products with a corn sweetener in them may lead to elevated inorganic mercury levels in your blood?
    _____
    _____
    _____

15. Which corn sweetener have you eaten the most of so far in your life?
    _____

16. How has the *type* of sugar being consumed by Americans changed since 1970 (Hint: see Table 4.4)?
    _____
    _____

17. Eating many products containing HFCS may lead to changes in the way some of your genes function. True or False

Food Colors and Heavy Metals

18. What must the package warning label on foods with yellow #5, red #40 and/or yellow #6 in them say In the European Union and United Kingdom?
    _____
    _____

19. Certified food colors in the U.S. and elsewhere may have allowable levels of lead, mercury, and arsenic in them.   True   or   False

European and US Food Color Research

20. Eating food products that contain certain food colors and/or sodium benzoate causes hyperactivity in children. True or False

21. Which of the following food colors have allowable mercury *or* lead residues? (Hint: Tables 4.5 and 4.6)

    a. Yellow 5
    b. Yellow 6
    c. Red 40
    d. Annatto
    e. Caramel
    f. all the above

22. The US has conducted all kinds of food color research.   True   or   False

Internet Research and Lead Exposures

23. Google: Do a keyword search on "ADHD and lead exposure." What did you find?
    _____
    _____

24. Certified food colors (Table 4.5) along with the less common food colors annatto, beta carotene, caramel, and titanium dioxide (Table 4.6) are all allowed to contain _____ppm lead.

25. List some preservatives that have allowable lead levels. _____, _____, _____, MSG, _____ and _____.

26. Sodium benzoate is a _____ with allowable impurities of _____ and _____.

27. Google. Do a keyword search on "autism and lead and mercury." What did you find?
    _____
    _____
    _____
    _____
    _____

28. Review: What is metallothionein and which gene is responsible for its production? What does it do for your body? What nutrient must you eat enough of to produce this important protein? (page 69 under US Food Color Research)

29. Click on each of the US Congressional Reports at the bottom of Dr. Dufault's Website: http://www.reneedufault.com/ Each report was written in 2021. As you read them, ask yourself *what is missing from these reports* based on what you learned in Chapter 4 of your textbook. What is not talked about in these reports? Write what you think here.

NOTE: Another way to access the Congressional reports below (if you are reading an e-book) is to simply click on the pictures and the link will open to the website.

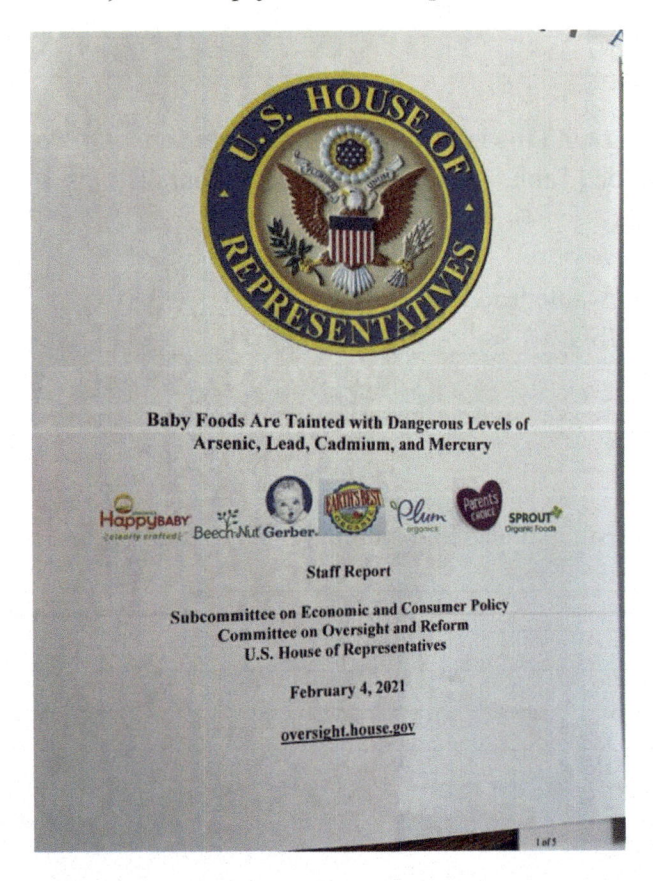

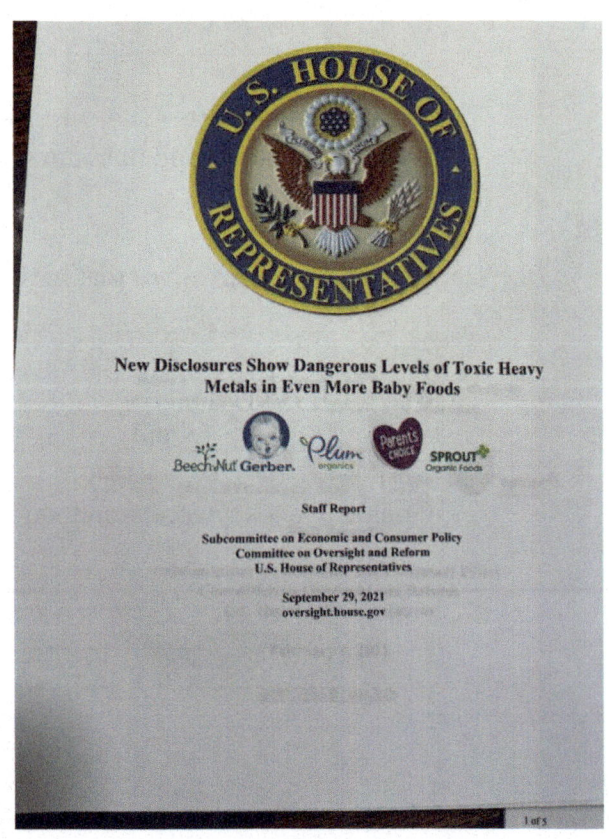

Nutritional Epigenetics: Unsafe at Any Meal Study Guide

Module 5

Our Western Diet and Disease

During this module of instruction, you will identify and evaluate changes in the western diet over the last forty years. You will learn how these changes have resulted in specific micronutrient deficiencies that have led to increases in neurodevelopmental disorders, type-2 diabetes, heart disease and other western disease conditions. American diet data will be used as a point of discussion.

LEARNING OBJECTIVES

1. Describe how the world's per capita refined sugar and vegetable consumption has changed over the last 40 years and how this change may impact health.

2. Recognize the factors that might explain the increasing inorganic blood mercury levels in the human population.

3. Explain how reductions in the intake of methyl donating and calcium rich foods can lead to adverse childbirth or health outcomes and increases in common western diseases (e.g., hypertension, heart disease, type-2 diabetes, Alzheimer's.)

4. Become familiar with recipes for preparing calcium rich meals.

5. Prepare and eat a calcium rich meal.

ACTIVITIES

1. As you read Chapter 5 of your textbook, complete the Chapter 5 Reading Guide provided in this study guide on pages 30-33.

2. View the United States Smithsonian Institute video titled "**Patterns of Health and Wellbeing: The Medicine of Food**" at the following link: https://www.si.edu/object/yt_IwapwKitM0k NOTE: The letters in bold (e.g. title of video) can be used in a Google or other search engine to find the video. In the space below provide your opinion of the video. What did you learn?

_____
_____
_____

3. Using Table 5.2 on page 88 of your textbook, find a healthy recipe that uses three of the calcium rich foods as ingredients. Use the recipe to prepare and eat a healthy calcium rich meal.

STUDY GROUP DISCUSSION QUESTIONS

- How has refined sugar consumption changed in the United States since 1970? What does this change mean in a population that is already magnesium deficient?

- What factors might explain the 29% decrease in American per capita consumption of calcium rich foods? What does this decrease mean for pregnancy and birth outcomes (e.g., lead detoxification, hypomethylation, low birth weight babies)?

- Share with a friend or study group partner the recipe you used to prepare a calcium rich meal. Was the meal tasty?

Need to find a healthy high calcium recipe? Try this one – Broccoli Cheese Soup

Ingredients: 2 tbsp. cold pressed olive oil, 1 medium white onion peeled and chopped, 3 garlic cloves peeled and chopped, 3 cups organic broccoli florets (can be fresh or frozen), 1 ½ cups organic milk, 1 ½ cups organic chicken or vegetable broth, ¼ tsp. pepper, ½ cup Greek yogurt (plain or honey), 1 1/2 – 2 cups grated white cheddar cheese.

Instructions: Sauté chopped garlic and onion in cold pressed olive oil on medium heat in a large pot. When vegetables soften, add broccoli florets, and mix gently. Cover the pot and cook the mixture on low heat for about ten minutes. Add organic broth to the mixture and then pour it into a blender. Mix on high speed until creamy. Pour mixture back into pot. Add in milk, pepper, and cheese. Stir on medium heat until cheese is melted, and mixture is hot. Stir in yogurt and serve.

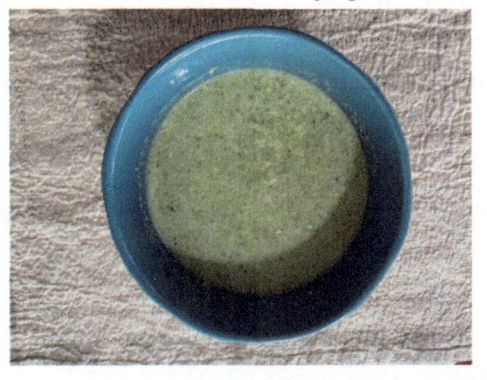

Healthy diet tip for today! Buy **cold pressed** or **cold extracted** "vegetable oils" as they are less likely to contain heavy metal residues because chemicals are not used in their manufacturing process. Olives, macadamia nuts, and sesame seeds are all fruits. When chemical processing aids are used to extract the oil from fruit seeds, there is a risk of heavy metal contamination. You want to reduce your heavy metal exposure to prevent neurological diseases such as Alzheimer's and Parkinson's.

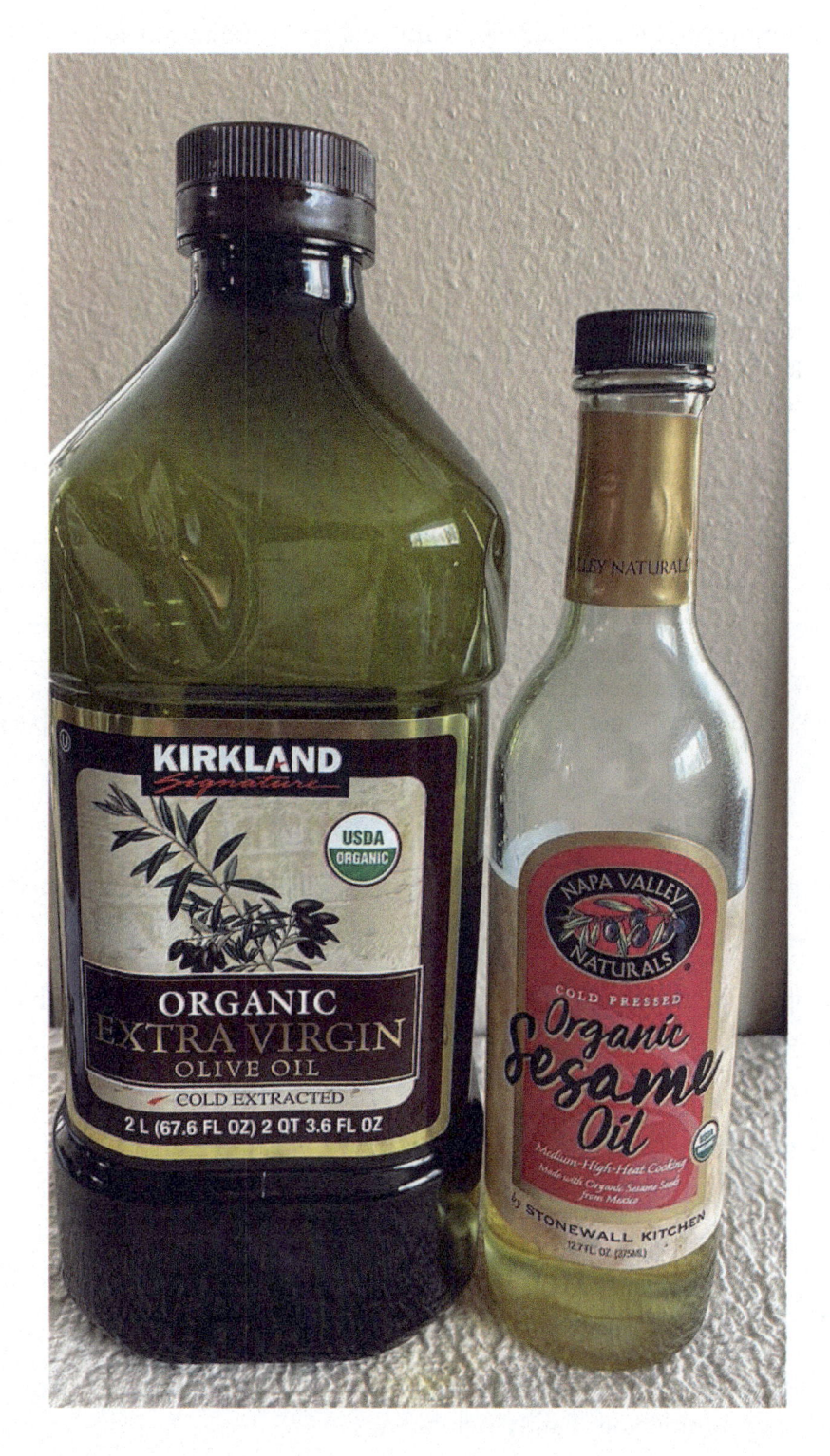

Reading Guide for Chapter 5, Module 5

Directions: Please answer the following questions as you are reading Chapter 5.

Standard American or Western Diet

1. How can what you eat either help or harm your body? (Hint: It has to do with genes.)
   _____
   _____
   _____

2. The SAD or "western diet" is characterized by eating which of the following:

   a. Refined grains
   b. Refined sugar or sweeteners
   c. Refined oils or fats
   d. All the above

Mexico

3. Mexico now has more obese citizens than the United States. Explain why this has occurred.
   _____
   _____
   _____

4. In 2014, the average American ate 46 pounds of high fructose corn syrup each year. True or False

China

5. Chinese officials are concerned about the rising daily intake or ingestion of _____ among the Chinese.

6. The adoption of the SAD by other countries has led to increases in which of the following health conditions:

   a. obesity
   b. diabetes
   c. vitamin deficiencies
   d. all the above

Unhealthy Diet Linked to Increasing Disease

7. Explain how obesity is a condition of *transgenerational* malnutrition and may impact future generations in your family's children.
   _____

_____
_____
_____

How the SAD Changes Your Physiology

8. The consumption of HFCS can lead to mineral imbalances or losses in human beings. True or False

Zinc Loss May Lead to Elevated Lead and Elevated Inorganic Blood Mercury Levels

9. What is the evidence to suggest that Americans are storing or bio-accumulating inorganic mercury in their blood?

_____
_____
_____
_____

10. Mercury is the only heavy metal exposure that increases your risk of heart disease and diabetes. True   False

Inorganic Blood Mercury Levels and Diabetes (Watch Smithsonian Video)

11. The Smithsonian presentation video makes it clear that type-2 diabetes is a result of _____ according to a study conducted at _____ community college.

12. Using the phrases in **BOLD**, complete the flow chart showing how diabetes can develop: **Consumption of foods containing HFCS, HFCS exposure, higher inorganic blood mercury levels, processed food consumption, diabetes diagnosis, higher fasting glucose (sugar) levels.**

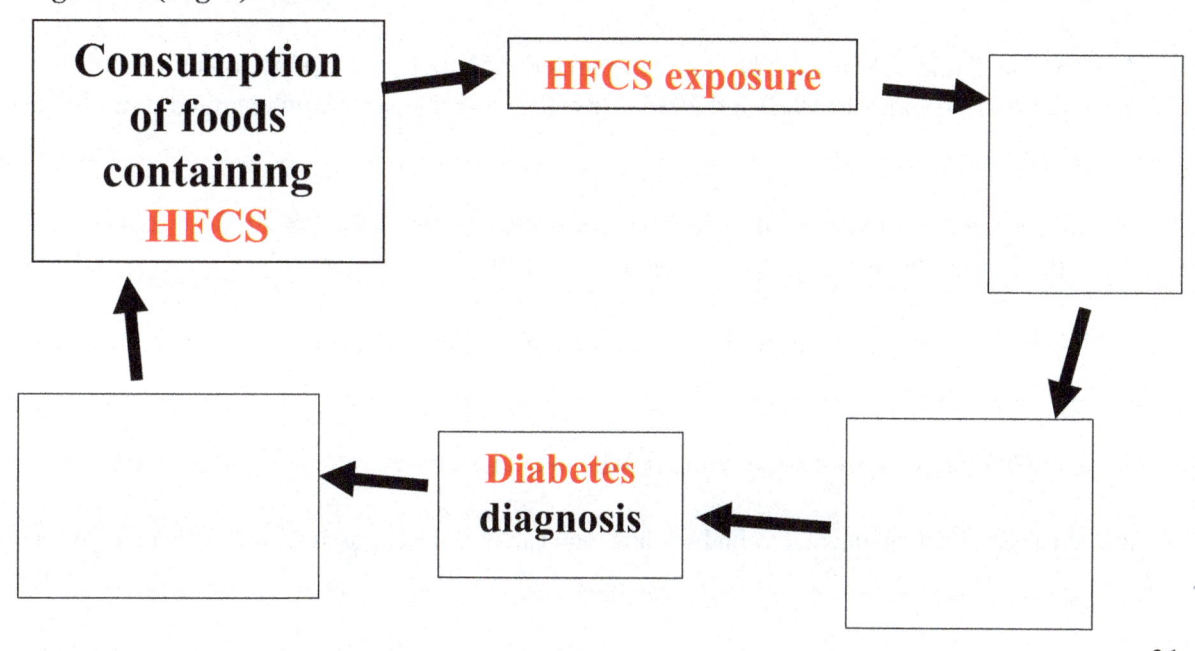

[Flow chart: **Consumption of foods containing HFCS** → **HFCS exposure** → [blank] → [blank] ← **Diabetes diagnosis** ← [blank] → (loop back to Consumption of foods containing HFCS)]

31

Dietary Deficits Add to Disease Risk

13. Magnesium deficiency is related to which of the following conditions:

    a. ADHD
    b. heart disease
    c. diabetes
    d. hypertension
    e. all the above

Calcium Deficit Problems in Children

14. When a person's dietary magnesium intake is low, and they are eating a lot of processed food that contains HFCS, they will become calcium deficient over time. True or False

15. Use the Internet to identify foods high in magnesium. Write your findings here:
    _____
    _____
    _____

16. Certain genes are dependent on calcium to function properly. They are _____ and _____.

17. What does the PON1 gene do for you?
    _____
    _____
    _____

18. The BDNF gene produces brain derived neurotrophic factor protein and this protein helps you keep your memories. True or False

19. Look at Table 5.2 on page 88 that compares the per person (capita) consumption of calcium rich foods in 1970 and 2012. How has milk consumption changed over the years?
    _____

20. The increased dietary intake of beverages sweetened with HFCS along with the overall reduction in dietary calcium are key factors in the development of _____ and ADHD.

21. What calcium rich foods could you see yourself eating more of?
    _____

22. Lead exposure is associated with ADHD and calcium deficiency. True or False

23. Do a search on the Internet to find out how you can become exposed to lead. What did you find?
    _____
    _____

Declines in Methyl-Donating Food Intake

24. Hypomethylation is when your body has too many methyl groups. True or False

25. What is a methyl group? (Hint: Refer to Chapter 2 of your book.)

26. Methyl groups are involved in making sure genes turn on and off properly. True or False

27. Hypomethylation is associated with which of the following disease conditions:

    a. autism
    b. Alzheimer's disease
    c. diabetes
    d. all the above

28. The following foods are high in both methyl groups and calcium:

    a. broccoli
    b. salmon
    c. milk
    d. spinach
    e. all the above

A Healthy Diet to Improve Your Health Status

29. With the information provided in Chapter 5, describe a healthy meal you would eat to improve your health status.

Brainstorming Notes

Use this space to write down your thoughts and ideas on what you can do with the information you are learning. As you become more knowledgeable about the role **food contaminants** (e.g. heavy metal and pesticide residues) play in the development of western disease, how can you share this new information with others?

Module 6

Spotlight on Autism and ADHD

During this module of instruction, we will discuss the increasing prevalence of autism and ADHD. The primary focus of this chapter will be on the United States where the education system is in crisis due to the increasing caseload of students requiring special education services. Since the textbook is older, an update will be provided in this workbook on the most recent prevalence data for autism and ADHD in the U.S. In this chapter, you will learn about the factors that contribute to the development of these debilitating neurodevelopmental disorders, which impact the quality of life and learning of a significant portion of the American population.

LEARNING OBJECTIVES

1. Recognize the role of diet in creating conditions for the development of autism and ADHD.

2. Describe the role of the PON1 gene in autism.

3. Explain the factors involved in PON1 gene expression (e.g., HFCS consumption, heavy metal exposure, dietary calcium deficits).

4. Recognize the symptoms of organophosphate pesticide poisoning.

5. Become familiar with food products listing the HFCS ingredient on the label and known to contain inorganic mercury residues.

ACTIVITIES

1. As you read Chapter 6 of your textbook, complete the Chapter 6 Reading Guide provided in this study guide on pages 40-43.

2. Visit the Institute for Agriculture and Trade Policy (IATP) website at the link provided and read the report titled, "**Not So Sweet: Missing Mercury and High Fructose Corn Syrup.**"

    https://www.iatp.org/sites/default/files/421_2_105026.pdf

Use Table 3 on page 14 of the IATP report to identify any of the food products containing HFCS and potential mercury residues that may be found in your own kitchen cupboards, freezer, and refrigerator. Of the seventeen products listed in Table 3, which did you find in your kitchen? How much mercury might you find in these products? Record your findings in the space below:

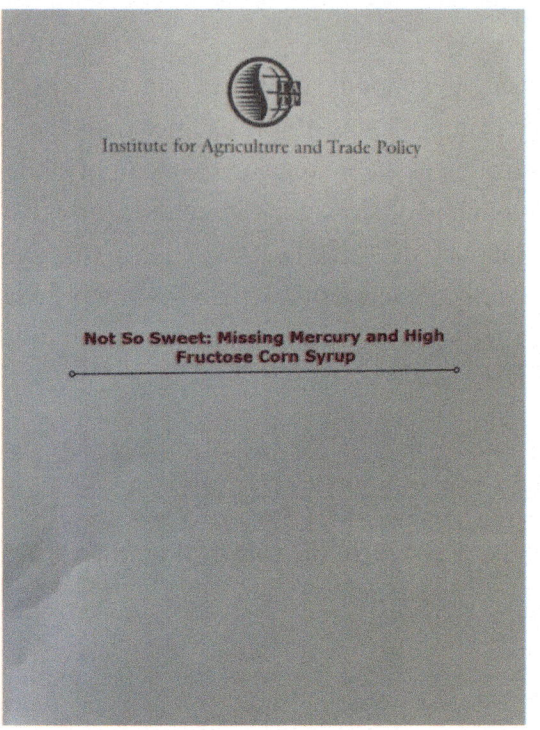

Institute for Agriculture and Trade Policy

Not So Sweet: Missing Mercury and High Fructose Corn Syrup

3. Your textbook was published in 2017. Are tools now available to connect heavy metal exposures to diet? Go to **PubMed** and look for the article titled, **Connecting inorganic mercury and lead levels in blood to dietary exposures.** This article was published in 2021. Read it in its entirety. Be prepared to discuss the role of the diet on the PON1 gene in autism and ADHD.

STUDY GROUP DISCUSSION QUESTIONS

- According to the IATP report and the material presented in Chapter 6 of your textbook, which food products have the highest mercury levels? Why would chocolate milk or baby formula be a significant source of inorganic mercury exposure?

  _____
  _____

- If you or a family member suffer from gastrointestinal distress or any of the other symptoms of organophosphate (OP) poisoning, what steps can you take to address the issue? Are their specific dietary changes that promote PON1 gene function to enhance the elimination of the OP pesticide residues you're your body?

- Based on the 2021 methodology article you read on PubMed, how can you determine if a child is exposed to heavy metals through diet? Is there a diet survey tool you can use to determine a child's eating pattern? Are there blood tests that can be conducted? After reading the article in its entirety, access the diet survey tool by clicking on this link: https://f6publishing.blob.core.windows.net/208175f9-e558-48cd-b3d7-6d41d6881e20/WJM-11-144-supplementary-material.pdf

    How can you use the diet survey tool to measure before and after changes in family diet?

2023 UPDATE ON AUTISM AND ADHD PREVALENCE IN AMERICA

On March 9, 2023, my colleagues and I published an article with an update on the prevalence of autism and ADHD in America. The article was published in the *World Journal of Clinical Pediatrics* and titled, Higher rates of autism and ADHD in American children: Are food quality issues impacting epigenetic inheritance? Read the title of the associated figure below (in bold) and then please **study** the figure:

Percentage distribution of American children receiving special education services, 2006 and 2021

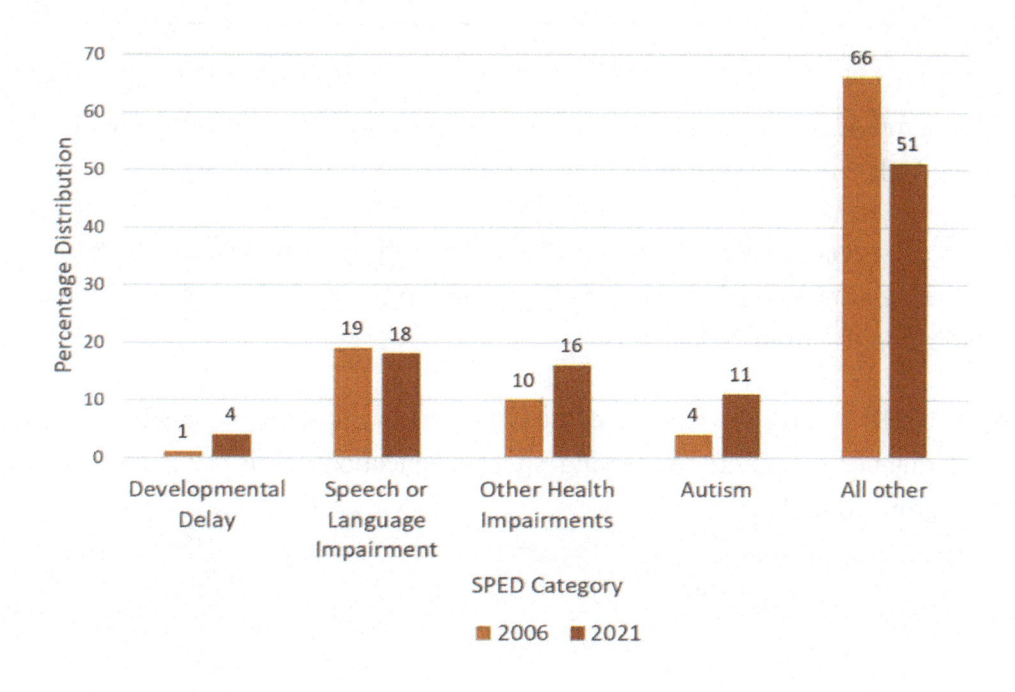

SPED Category	2006	2021
Developmental Delay	1	4
Speech or Language Impairment	19	18
Other Health Impairments	10	16
Autism	4	11
All other	66	51

Dr. Renee Joy Dufault

BAR CHART INTERPRETATION:

- There are a total of 13 disability categories in the U.S. under which students may qualify for special education services. The bar chart on the previous page (37) shows data for four outstanding categories including developmental delay, speech or language, other health impairments, and autism; the remaining nine categories are lumped together as "all other." The four outstanding categories are those under which children with autism and/or ADHD may receive services.

- Another way of looking at the bar chart, is to see that in 2006, 34% of children receiving special education services were receiving them for autism and/or ADHD related disabilities. By 2021, 49%, or nearly half, of all the children receiving special education services were receiving them for autism and/or ADHD related disabilities.

Now read the title (in bold) below and **study** this table:

Number of U.S. students ages 6-21 served under Individuals with Disabilities Education Act by disability category & year.

Year	Autism	OHI (Including ADHD)	Speech/ Language	Developmental Delay (3-9 yrs. only)	All Disabilities
2006	224,594	599,494	1,160,904	89,931	6,081,890
2021	768,179	1,097,251	1,183,310	255,787	6,712,010
%Change (2006-2021)	+242.0 %	+ 83.0 %	+1.9%	+ 184.4%	+10.4 %

- While student enrollment in U.S. schools remains relatively flat, the percentage of children receiving special education services overall increased 10.4% from 2006-2021.

- The categories of special education services that include those provided to children with autism show the highest caseload increases with autism increasing 242% and developmental delay increasing 184.4% from 2006-2021.

- Children with ADHD receive services under the Other Heath Impairments special education category. The number of children receiving special education services in this category increased 83% from 2006-2021.

Now read the title (in bold) below and **study** this figure of U.S. student enrollment provided to me by the U.S. Department of Education:

Actual and projected numbers for enrollment in U.S. elementary and secondary schools, by grade level: Fall 2003 through Fall 2028.

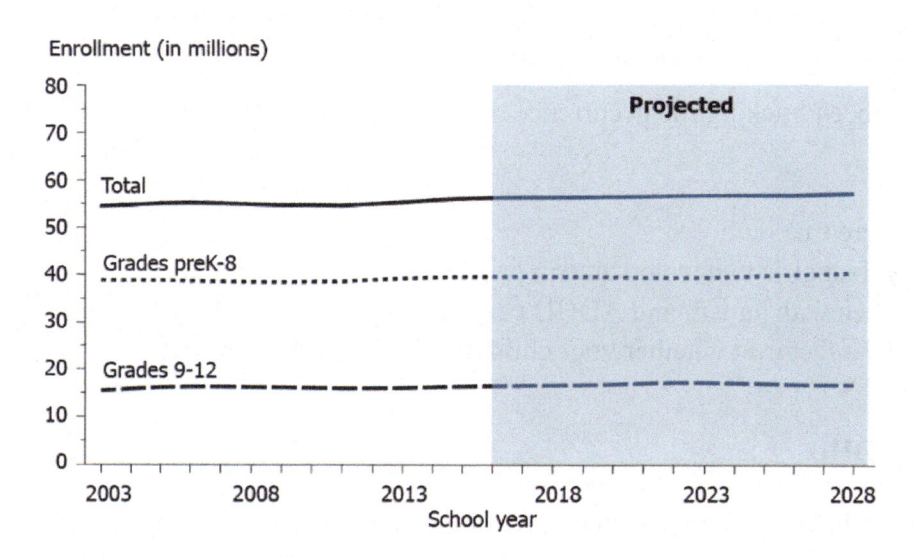

Now **read** the following:

Abstract

In the United States, schools offer special education services to children who are diagnosed with a learning or neurodevelopmental disorder and have difficulty meeting their learning goals. Pediatricians may play a key role in helping children access special education services. The number of children ages 6-21 in the United States receiving special education services increased 10.4% from 2006 to 2021. Children receiving special education services under the autism category increased 242% during the same period. The demand for special education services for children under the developmental delay and other health impaired (OHI) categories increased by 184% and 83% respectively. Although student enrollment in American schools has remained stable since 2006, the percentage distribution of children receiving special education services nearly tripled for the autism category and quadrupled for the developmental delay category by 2021. Allowable heavy metal residues remain persistent in the American food supply due to food ingredient manufacturing processes. Numerous clinical trial data indicate heavy metal exposures and poor diet are the primary epigenetic factors responsible for the autism and attention deficit hyperactivity disorder epidemics. **Dietary heavy metal exposures, especially inorganic mercury and lead may impact gene behavior across generations**. In 2021, the United States Congress found heavy metal residues problematic in the American food supply but took no legislative action. Mandatory health warning labels on select foods may be the only way to reduce dietary heavy metal exposures and improve child learning across generations.

Dr. Renee Joy Dufault

Reading Guide for Chapter 6, Module 6

Directions: Please answer the following questions as you are reading Chapter 6.

Increasing Prevalence of Autism and ADHD

1. The word "prevalence" means the same thing as the word _____.

2. The CDC in the US has been tracking the occurrence of autism and ADHD since _____.

3. Which of the following are true:
   a. Boys are more likely than girls to develop autism or ADHD
   b. The numbers of children with autism and ADHD continue to climb in the U.S.
   c. Where you live can be a factor in whether your child develops autism or ADHD
   d. all the above

Root Causes of Autism and ADHD

4. Common factors in the development of autism and ADHD include exposure to _____ (heavy metals or calcium?) and pesticides.

Pesticide Exposure is a Risk Factor

5. The pesticide exposure most connected to the development of autism and ADHD is
   a. malathion
   b. organophosphate (OP) pesticides
   c. both a and b

6. When a child with ADHD switches to an organic diet, what will happen? Name two things.
   _____
   _____

7. Prenatal pesticide exposures may occur in a woman's _____. (Hint: Where a child comes from.)

8. DD means _____ _____.

9. When pregnant women live near agriculture fields where farmers apply pesticides, they are more likely to have poor birth outcomes.   True   or   False

PON1 Gene Expression Suppressors

10. The availability and activity of the PON1 enzyme is impaired in children with _____ and _____.

40

Nutritional Epigenetics: Unsafe at Any Meal Study Guide

11. Families need to avoid eating foods with the ingredients _____ and _____ to prevent calcium losses in their bodies.

12. Factors that change the way the PON1 gene works include which of the following:
    a. alcohol
    b. fructose including HFCS
    c. inorganic mercury
    d. lead
    e. all the above

13. IF you do not reduce your processed food consumption, what heavy metal(s) may increase in your blood? _____

14. Inorganic mercury suppresses (dampens) PON1 gene activity leaving you vulnerable to the toxic impacts of organophosphate pesticide exposures. True or False

PON1 Gene Expression in Children

15. Age is the most important factor of all when it comes to _____ gene activity. In children before birth and for several years after birth, PON1 gene activity is very _____. This means children are not as able to produce the enzyme required to break down OP Pesticide residues.

16. To help children achieve the very best health and learning outcomes, the family diet should be free of
_____

What does OP pesticide exposure and poisoning look like?

17. Children with low PON1 gene activity may show many different symptoms. List four of them. _____, _____, _____, and _____.

Obesity Issues pg. 104-108

18. Maternal obesity increases the risk of bearing a child with autism or ADHD. True or False

19. Tunnel vision is why scientists have not solved many of the chronic disease problems. True or False

20. What does "tunnel vision" mean when it comes to science?
_____
_____

21. HFCS consumption in the US by women may be a factor in the development of which of the following:

41

a. obesity
b. the rate of autism
c. Children becoming obese adults
d. Children developing high blood pressure and heart disease
e. all the above

22. In addition to avoiding sugar and HFCS during pregnancy, women can prevent babies from becoming obese by not feeding their babies _____ _____.

23. Google using the following key words, "baby formula and heavy metals." What did you find?
_____
_____

24. Why might baby formulas contain heavy metal residues? (Hint: Look at ingredient label).
_____
_____

Autism and ADHD Prevention or Treatment

25. What can parents do to bring about positive changes in their child's behavior and health?
_____
_____

26. Poor diet continues to play a role in autism and ADHD. True or False

27. The younger a child with ADHD or autism, the better chance he/she has of healing through healthy diet. True or False

28. A child with ADHD or autism is genetically prone to these conditions and must always avoid eating highly processed foods that contain substances that may become toxic over time with bioaccumulation. True or False

Medication

29. Doctors are trained to teach parents about healthy diet. True or False

30. Only _____ percent of medical schools require their students to take a nutrition course.

31. Why would a parent put their child on medication without trying dietary changes first?
_____
_____

32. What are some problems that may crop up with the use of medication over time?
_____

Prevention vs Treatment Tools

33. In 2021, there was an article published to provide guidance on determining if diet contributes to inorganic mercury and lead exposures in children with symptoms of autism or ADHD. That article provides a link to a supplementary page that you can access to find a helpful tool. What is that tool? (Hint: Click on link to supplementary page)
   _____

34. In your opinion what should be done to prevent autism or ADHD in your community's children?
   _____
   _____

35. How might a child with autism or ADHD suffer though out his/her life?
    a. S/he may be at increased risk of obesity
    b. S/he may be at increased risk of heart disease as an adult
    c. S/he may have difficulty learning in school
    d. S/he may get into trouble and become a youth offender
    e. S/he may become physically or mentally disabled over time due to the side effects of medication
    f. Any of the above

36. **Study** the figure below. Hg = mercury, Pb = lead, Ca = calcium, Zn = zinc.

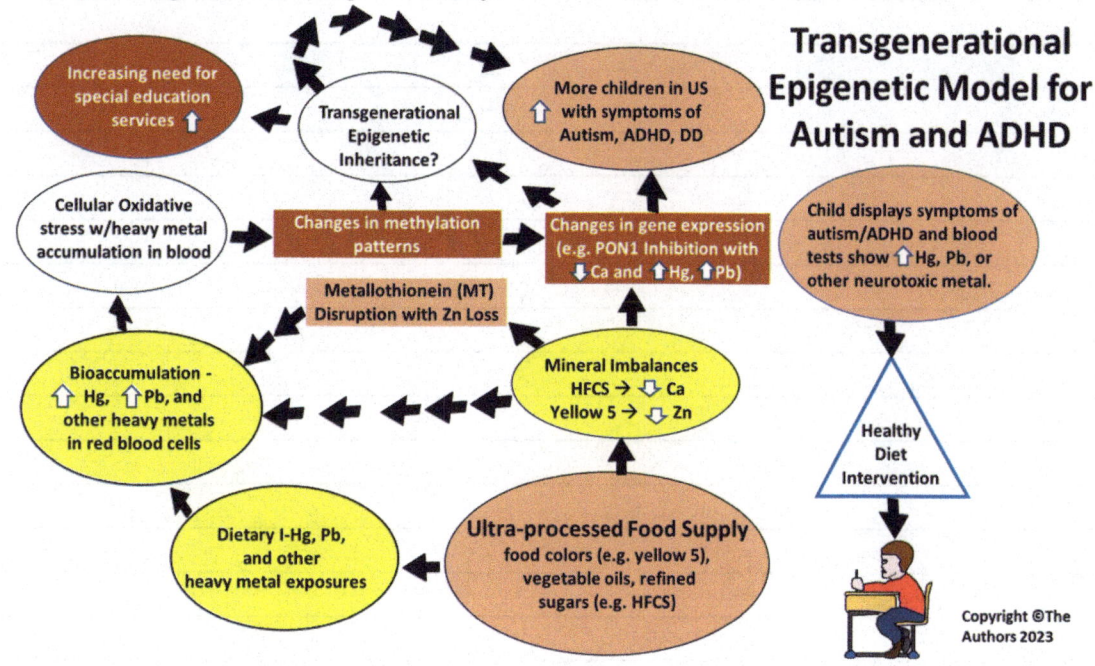

Brainstorming Notes

Use this space to write down your thoughts and ideas on what you can do with the information you are learning. As you become more knowledgeable about the root causes of autism and ADHD, how can you share this new information with others?

Module 7

Food Labeling Practices

During this module of instruction, you will learn about the regulations pertaining to food ingredient safety and labeling and the marketing strategies food manufacturers use to sell their food and supplement products. You will learn how to make healthier choices as you shop for groceries.

LEARNING OBJECTIVES

1. Describe the regulatory process involved in determining whether a food ingredient is "safe."

2. Explain how food ingredient labels can be used by the consumer to determine a product's safety.

3. Recognize the role of marketing in the development of unhealthy dietary patterns.

4. Explain how the use of supplements can be a risky dietary behavior.

5. Recognize why one product may be a healthier choice compared to another.

ACTIVITIES

1. As you read Chapter 7 of your textbook, complete the Chapter 7 Reading Guide provided in this study guide on pages 48-51.

2. Watch the Ted Talk at the following link that discusses the current food marketing practices aimed at children. **Marketing food to children - Anna Lappe** (If you can't click on the link provided, please use the title of the video in a key word search). After watching the video, write your reflection in the space below:

Reflect on how marketing practices may have influenced your dietary pattern or food choices over the years. What if anything, could have been done to counterbalance the marketing to enable you to adopt healthier eating habits?

_____
_____
_____

3. Survey your kitchen and identify food products that may contain misleading information on the packaging due to marketing practices. Also identify any products that contain any of the GRAS ingredients listed in **Table 7.1 on page 120** of your textbook. The products that contain those GRAS ingredients may contain allowable heavy metal impurities. Use the table below to list the products you found in your kitchen that have misleading labels or GRAS ingredients.

Product	Misleading information? (specify)	GRAS ingredient on label?? (specify)

STUDY GROUP DISCUSSION QUESTIONS

- Review the food products you listed in the table on the previous page (46). Discuss ways you can eliminate these food products from your diet. What are some healthier alternatives to these products? Instead of buying the product, could you make it from scratch using single ingredient foods?

  _____
  _____
  _____

- Discuss the risks and the benefits of taking supplements or eating gluten free foods (if you do not have celiac disease).

  _____
  _____
  _____

- Considering the marketing and labeling practices of food manufacturers, what can you do to protect yourself from misinformation? See gluten free water and gluten free juice pops below. Would you expect wheat to be found in water or juice?

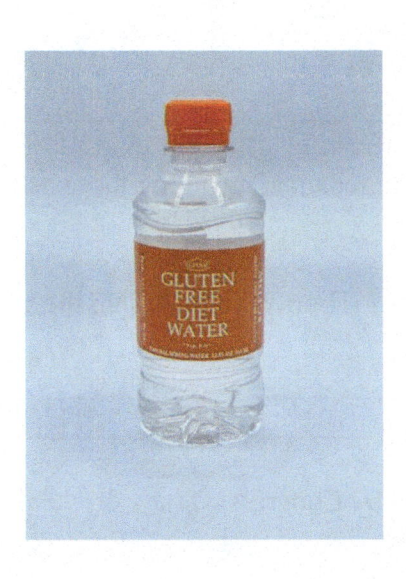

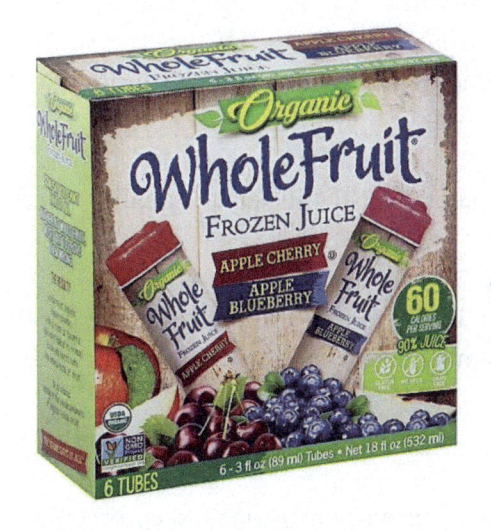

  _____
  _____
  _____

Dr. Renee Joy Dufault

Reading Guide for Chapter 7, Module 7

Directions: Please answer the following questions as you are reading Chapter 7.

Introduction

1. Food labels are deceptive in their marketing. What does this mean? Define the word deceptive in relation to food labeling.
   _____
   _____

Establishing the FDA

2. Which of the following are true about the 1906 Pure Food and Drug Act enacted by the US Congress:
   a. The Act was passed in response to Sinclair's book about the meat packing industry
   b. A goal of the Act was to ban food ingredients that would be harmful to health.
   c. The intent of Congress was to establish a consumer agency that would regulate product labeling in terms of accuracy.
   d. The intent of Congress was to prevent misbranding and misrepresenting what a product can do
   e. all the above

FDA and USP's Roles in Ingredient Safety

3. Prior to 1906, there was no FDA or food safety regulatory agency. Instead, there was the _____.

4. The US Pharmacopeial Convention (USP) began setting standards for drug and ingredient quality in _____.

5. Name four ingredients in use during the 1800's.
   _____

6. Today the USP still sets the quality standards for all ingredients, including those used in food products. True or False

7. The USP is a trade organization. What does that mean? (Hint: Who makes up the USP? Membership?)
   _____
   _____

8. FDA's primary mission is to enforce the laws adopted by Congress. True or False

9. Where does the FDA get its safety standards for food ingredients?

10. Where does the responsibility for food ingredient safety ultimately lie? Who is ensuring food ingredients are made according to the recommended safety standards?

The GRAS Process

11. Prior to the 1950's, there were few standards for food ingredient safety.   True   or   False

12. In 1958, Congress amended the Pure Food and Drug Act by passing the Food Additives Amendment.   True   or   False

13. The Food Additives Amendment required food manufacturers to

14. In 1958, FDA grandfathered a bunch of food ingredients into the category "Generally Recognized as Safe" even though none of the ingredients had undergone any safety testing.   True   or   False

15. Today if you want to add a food ingredient to the Generally Recognized as Safe list then you must submit a petition to the _____.

How HFCS was determined as "safe"

16. In 1983, FDA approved the corn refining industry's petition to consider HFCS a GRAS substance for which of the following reasons:
    a. HFCS is made using an enzyme already considered GRAS by FDA
    b. HFCS is a little like honey,
    c. HFCS is a little like corn syrup and corn sugar, both GRAS by the FDA
    d. All the above

17. As to the harm caused by HFCS to "sensitive populations," FDA reviewers wrote that the requirement to list HFCS on the ingredient label was

18. What did FDA do about HFCS in 1996 in response to objections from a diabetes research center?

GRAS Database

19. When a substance has GRAS status it can be added to foods without _____.

20. There are hundreds of GRAS substances used as food ingredients in the food supply.   True   or   False

21. Some GRAS substances have allowable heavy metal residues.   True   or   False

22. From Table 7.1, name two food ingredients you have seen on food ingredient labels along with their allowable heavy metal levels. _____ and _____.

Food Labeling Requirements

23. FDA preapproves each food label before it goes on a food package.   True   or   False

24. Food ingredients must be listed on the food label according to how much of the ingredient is in the product with the first ingredient indicating what the product is mostly made up of.   True   or   False

25. In the following label, which ingredient is the food mostly made up of? (circle)

    INGREDIENTS: Whole wheat flour, water, high fructose corn syrup, corn syrup, egg, soybean oil, sugar

26. Trace amounts of heavy metals do not have to be listed on the food ingredient label.   True   or   False

27. Organic foods are the same thing as natural foods.   True or False

28. A highly processed food can still carry the "natural" label.   True   or   False

Food Marketing Practices

29. Gluten-free marketing is used to sell foods that do not even contain wheat, barley or rye grains that contain gluten proteins. For example, bottled water can be sold as gluten free. As a consumer, what do you think about this practice?
    _____
    _____

30. Why would food manufacturers place a "gluten free" label on their food product when there is no chance the product could even contain gluten?
    _____

31. Do a Google search on the key words "gluten free and mercury exposure." What did you find?
    _____
    _____

The Problem with Eating Gluten-Free

32. Eating a gluten free diet can lead to nutrient deficiency. List some nutrients you may not get enough of if you eat a gluten free diet.
   _____
   _____
   _____

33. A gluten allergy presents with a set of symptoms that are very much like the symptoms of OP pesticide exposure.   True   or   False

34. Children with autism have low PON1 gene activity and thus have difficulty breaking down OP pesticide residues. They often have symptoms of OP pesticide poisoning which are the same as the symptoms of _____ allergy.

Supplements

35. Supplement use may be dangerous for which of the following reasons:
    a. benefits and risks are unknown
    b. co-exposure to a variety of supplements could result in liver injury
    c. some supplements can actually increase your risk of heart attack
    d. all the above

36. Google "supplement use and CVD." What did you find?
   _____
   _____
   _____

Conclusion

37. The safest product to buy is one made with _____ ingredients as well as with the _____ amount of ingredients.

CHALLENGE QUESTION: From what you've learned thus far from your studies, what makes pepperoni pizza unhealthy? Think about the ingredients and possible heavy metal and pesticide residues. _____

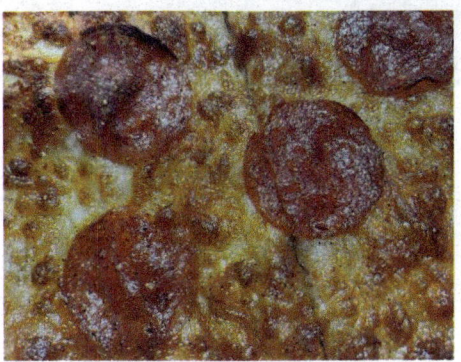

51

STUDY THIS FOOD PYRAMID

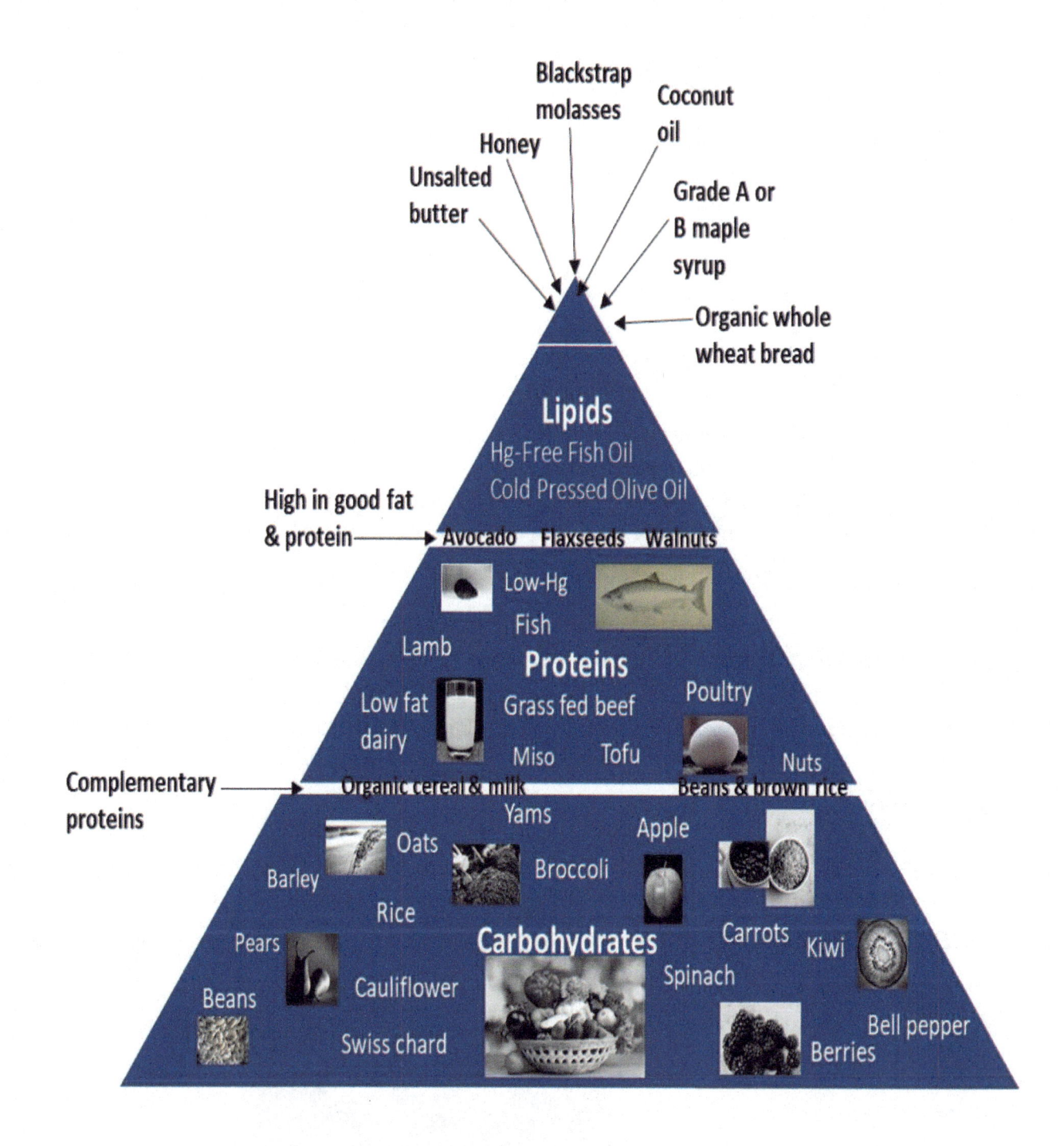

Top of pyramid (use sparingly):
- Unsalted butter
- Honey
- Blackstrap molasses
- Coconut oil
- Grade A or B maple syrup
- Organic whole wheat bread

Lipids
- Hg-Free Fish Oil
- Cold Pressed Olive Oil

High in good fat & protein → Avocado, Flaxseeds, Walnuts

Proteins
- Low-Hg Fish
- Lamb
- Low fat dairy
- Grass fed beef
- Poultry
- Miso
- Tofu
- Nuts

Complementary proteins → Organic cereal & milk, Beans & brown rice

Carbohydrates
- Barley
- Oats
- Yams
- Apple
- Pears
- Rice
- Broccoli
- Carrots
- Kiwi
- Beans
- Cauliflower
- Spinach
- Swiss chard
- Berries
- Bell pepper

Module 8

Creating a Safe Food Environment

During this final module of instruction, you will learn about the three macromolecules required to maintain good health and how to obtain them safely from the current food supply. You will learn how to create a healthy food environment in your home.

LEARNING OBJECTIVES

1. Become familiar with the three major macromolecules the body needs to thrive and how to obtain them from the current food supply.

2. Explain whether Americans are meeting their dietary recommendations for fats (lipids), carbohydrates, and proteins.

3. Recognize how excessive fructose intake can lead to fatty liver disease over time.

4. Describe foods high in protein and zinc and understand their role in healthy gene function.

5. Recognize the changes you can make to ensure a safe and healthy food environment in your home.

ACTIVITIES

1. As you read Chapter 8 of your textbook, complete the Chapter 8 Reading Guide provided in this study guide on pages 55-58.

2. Do a keyword search on the Internet using the term "fructose and fatty liver disease." Read articles of interest to you or view videos. Your textbook was published in 2017. Is there additional evidence to show that over-consumption of high fructose corn syrup may lead to fatty liver disease? Discuss two new things you learned from your research.

_____
_____
_____
_____
_____
_____
_____

3. Survey your kitchen cupboards, refrigerator and freezer to identify foods that are both high in zinc and protein. Use Table 8.1 on page 140 of your textbook as a reference for identifying foods high in both zinc and protein. Report you survey findings in the table below:

Foods found in my kitchen that are high in both zinc and protein

STUDY GROUP DISCUSSION QUESTIONS

- From reading chapter 8, discuss whether you think your dietary intake of lipids, carbohydrates, and proteins meet the healthy guidelines provided in your textbook. Are you eating enough healthy fat, such as foods high omega-3 (pg. 136 of your textbook)? Are you eating enough good carbs (pg. 146 of your textbook)? Healthy protein?

- How has your food environment changed at home over the last eight weeks? Have you eliminated unhealthy food products from your kitchen? Have you learned how to create a healthy food environment in your home? Discuss any changes you've made.

Reading Guide for Chapter 8, Module 8

Directions: Please answer the following questions as you are reading Chapter 8.

Healthy Diet Guidelines

1. Check out the food pyramid I created on pg. 133 of your book. What is missing from the pyramid?
   _____

2. Carbohydrates can be good or bad. Give an example of a good carb. _____
   Give an example of a bad carb. _____

3. Lipids are fats. There are foods high in fat that are good for you. See my pyramid. What are healthy sources of good fat? Provide three examples. _____, _____, and _____.

4. Look at the top of the pyramid? What do you see at the top? _____, _____, _____, _____ are all examples of foods you should eat only in small amounts. Foods with these ingredients are "treats."

Comparing Food Pyramids Released by US Government

5. Conduct internet research to find some of the food pyramids used by the US Department of Agriculture (USDA) over the years. See one of them below: How do these pyramids differ from the one I provide on pg. 133 of your textbook?

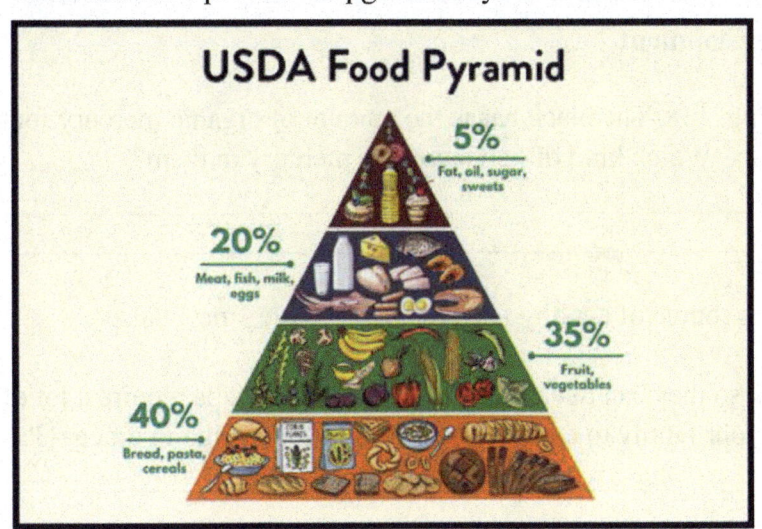

   Please provide your thoughts on the guidance you have been given by the US government through the years on what to eat.
   _____
   _____

Lipids (Fats)

6. Dietary fats are important sources of _____ and they also provide the materials to build the fat _____ around each cell in your body.

7. The primary function of the cell membrane is to control the flow of _____ in and out of cells.

8. Unsaturated fats are great for health sustainability. Name the two most important unsaturated fats you can eat. _____ and _____.

9. Omega-3 fats can be found in a variety of foods. Look at the list on pg. 136. Which of these foods can you eat more of?
   _____
   _____

10. Saturated (bad) fats are commonly found in what kind of food? See list on pg. 135. (Hint: The food is not slow.)
    _____

11. Eating less saturated fat and not eating any _____ fat will improve your health profile especially if you increase your intake of healthy omega-3 fats.

12. What do foods high in saturated and trans-fat have in common? See lists on pg. 135.
    _____

Mercury in Fish and Child Development

13. Look at the bar chart on pg. 138. The black bar is the amount of organic mercury found in different fish and shellfish. Which kind of fish have less mercury in them?
    _____
    _____

14. Salmon looks like a great source of healthy fat (omega-3). True or False

15. Children need healthy fat so they can develop good brains. Brain cells require a lot of fat. What would you advise your family to eat when it comes to foods high in omega-3?
    _____
    _____

Proteins

16. Which of the following jobs do proteins do in your body?
    a. They transport sugar and other nutrients in and out of your cells.
    b. They serve as antibodies for your immune system so you can fight infection.
    c. They contribute the blocks needed to build new proteins in your body.
    d. They transport heavy metals out of your body.
    e. They serve as glue for sticking memories in your brain.
    f. all the above

17. An amino acid is the same thing as a _____.

18. What is a zinc finger and what does it do?
    _____
    _____

19. Table 8.1 on page 140 of your textbook provides a list of foods rich in protein and zinc. List your favorites.
    _____
    _____

20. What are the children in the US eating when it comes to protein? Hint: See Grimes study findings and then describe some of the issues.
    _____
    _____

Carbohydrates

21. Carbohydrates provide your body with glucose which is needed to _____ and
    _____.

22. Fructose is a carbohydrate that is never naturally occurring. True or False

23. Fructose is not needed by the human body. Over eating fructose can lead to
    _____
    _____.

24. Fatty liver disease not created by drinking too much alcohol is called
    _____.

25. Almost one quarter or 25% of the American population is suffering from NAFLD. True or False

26. There are good carbs and bad carbs. High intake of bad carbs leads to which disease conditions?

Additional Suggestions

27. Of the suggestions I provide at the bottom of pg. 147 and top of page 148, which can you follow easily?

28. How can you reduce your pesticide exposures even if you do not have access to organic foods?

29. What you eat or do not eat is your body's only defense against disease.   True   or   False

30. Congratulations! You have completed your LAST reading guide!!!!! How do you feel?

ANSWER KEY TO READING GUIDES

Chapter 1, Module 1

1. True   2. 200 ppm   3. Liver, heart   4. False   5. d, all the above

6. True   7. True   8. True   9. Contaminated with lead, overconsumption   10. Upper

11. True   12. True   13. Buildup of toxicant in tissues   14. Decreased   15. Yes, not safe.

16. may be different in each state   17. True   18. False   19. Calcium

20. Inability to differentiate between smells   21. c, all the above   22. Recognized, safe

23. True   24. Organic   25. Autism, ADHD, diabetes, and other   26. Gene

27. chlorine, hydrogen chloride, sodium hydroxide   28. True   29. 1 ppm   30. True

31. 36 pounds   32. Blood, hair, fingernails, urine

33. Consumed in amounts higher than your body can excrete

Chapter 2, Module 2

1. True   2. True   3. Liver cells breakdown toxicants, blood cells fight bacterial infection

4. Methylation   5. Nucleus   6. Cell differentiation   7. d, all the above   8. Epigenetics

9. True   10. False   11. e, all the above   12. True   13. True   14. Food

15. choline, folic acid, folate, methionine   16. Individual response   17. Individual response

18. oncogenes   19. d, all the above   20. Tumor suppressor   21. Diet, nutrition   22. True

23. See completed table below:

Short name (acronym)	Long name (protein)	Your body uses this protein to _____.
MT	metallothionein	Carry and excrete metals
BDNF	Brain derived neurotrophic factor	attach memories to brain cells.
PON1	Paraoxonase-1	breaks down pesticide residues

24. Calcium, individual responses based on internet search   25. Calcium   26. a. liver

27. e, all the above   28. Zinc   29. Alzheimer's, ADHD   30. Metals bioaccumulate

31. HDL

Chapter 3, Module 3

1. True   2. EPA, disinfectant, fungicide   3. True   4. True

5. chlorine   6. False   7. d, all the above   8. True   9. d, all the above

10. Yes   11. True   12. False   13. Vegetables, wheat   14. Individual responses

15. from label on page 49 of textbook – **heavy metal exposures** from red 40, blue 2, yellow 6, annatto, blue 1, vegetable oil and **pesticide exposures** from corn flour, wheat flour, whole grain oat flour

16. YES and No…. Zhou et al. (2019) did develop a mouse model that can now be used as a human model to determine the adverse effects of DIETARY co-exposures to inorganic mercury, lead, and cadmium.

17. True   18. d, both a and b   19. False   20. True   21. Individual responses

22. keep organic flour in the refrigerator to preserve and protect against mold and bug infestations

23. Individual response

Chapter 4, Module 4

1. e, all the above   2. True   3. The bioaccumulation of heavy metals in blood increase risk of chronic diseases (obesity, diabetes, heart disease).

4. False   5. FEDIOL, is the European Union (EU) vegetable oil trade organization that published a risk assessment for contaminants found in vegetable oils.

6. True   7. American vegetable (cooking oil) consumption increased 250% between 1970-2010.

8. True   9. d, all the above   10. Heart, diabetes   11. Mercuric chloride   12. True

13. f, all the above   14. Dufault et al., (2015) Fort Peck Study   15. Individual response

16. HFCS consumption increased 8,833%   17. True   18. "*May have an adverse effect on activity and attention in children.*"

19. True   20. True   21. f, all the above   22. False   23. Lead exposure likely cause of ADHD

24. 10 ppm   25. Table 4.7   26. Preservative, lead and mercury   27. Lead and mercury exposure a likely cause of autism

28. Metallothionein is a zinc dependent metal transporter protein that prevents the build up of heavy metals in your body.

29. U.S. Congressional reports do not look at heavy metal residues in foods eaten by children and adults.

Chapter 5, Module 5

1. Diet determines gene behavior for better or worse. Poor diet makes you more susceptible to disease because your body cannot metabolize and excrete harmful agents that cause disease.

2. d, all the above   3. In 1994, the NAFTA trade agreement ensured that Mexico could buy HFCS and other ingredients found in highly processed foods. Consumption of highly processed foods increased dramatically in Mexico, and this increased the obesity prevalence.

4. True   5. Vegetable oils   6. d, all the above   7. As an obese expectant mother consumes HFCS (an obesogenic), she will experience nutritional deficits and give birth to a child who is metabolically programmed to become obese.

8. True   9. Dan Laks analyzed blood sample results collected by the CDC from 1999-2006 and found the older a woman becomes; the higher the inorganic mercury levels will be in her blood.

10. False   11. Inorganic mercury accumulation, Fort Peck   12. See diagram below:

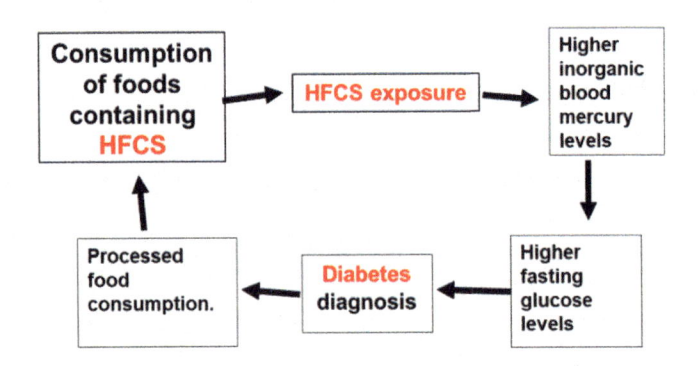

Consumption of foods containing HFCS → HFCS exposure → Higher inorganic blood mercury levels → Higher fasting glucose levels → Diabetes diagnosis → Processed food consumption → (back to Consumption of foods containing HFCS)

13. e, all the above   14. True   15. Individual responses   16. BDNF, PON1

17. PON1 provides the instructions for making paraoxonase enzyme which your body needs to detoxify organophosphate pesticide residues

18. True   19. Decreased   20. Autism   21. Individual responses   22. True

23. Individual responses   24. False   25. One carbon attached to three hydrogen atoms

26. True   27. d, all the above   28. e, all the above   29. Individual responses

Chapter 6, Module 6

1. occurrence   2. 2000   3. d, all the above   4. Heavy metals   5. c, both a and b

6. lowered exposure to OP pesticide residues and reduction in ADHD symptoms

7. womb   8. Developmental delay   9. True   10. Autism, ADHD   11. fructose, HFCS

12. e, all the above   13. Inorganic blood mercury   14. True   15. PON1, low

16. contaminants that may suppress PON1 gene activity   17. See top of page 104 in textbook

18. True   19. True   20. Lack of interdisciplinary research or a focus on single theories

21. e, all the above   22. Baby formula   23. Baby formula is often contaminated with heavy metals

24. Table 6.1 page 107 of textbook   25. Adopt a healthy diet free of pesticide and heavy metal residues   26. True   27. True   28. True   29. False   30. 25%   31. Ignorance, Ritalin

32. drug abuse, heart attack, stroke, see list on page 111 of textbook

33. diet survey form   34. Individual responses   35. f, all the above

Chapter 7, Module 7

1. Labels omit trace contaminants and processing aid chemicals.   2. e, all the above   3. USP

4. 1820   5. Tonics, extracts, syrups, vinegars   6. True

7. The US Pharmacopeial Convention (USP) is made up of members who represent and are working for the regulated industries.

8. True   9. The FDA gets its safety standards for food ingredients from the USP.

10. The responsibility for food ingredient safety lies with the food manufacturers.   11. True
12. True   13. Determine the safety of food ingredients   14. True   15. FDA

16. d, all the above   17. Warning enough   18. FDA reaffirmed its decision to consider HFCS GRAS

19. restriction   20. True   21. True   22. See Table 7.1, page 120 of your textbook.

23. False   24. True   25. Whole wheat flour   26. True   27. False   28. True

29. Individual response   30. Mo money   31. Mercury exposure is higher with greater consumption of gluten free foods

32. Numerous studies show lower protein, folate, calcium, vitamin D intakes are associated with gluten free diet

33. True   34. Gluten   35. d, all the above   36. Higher risk of CVD with supplement use

37. organic, least

38. Pepperoni pizza may contain pesticide residues if the crust is made from conventional flour; heavy metal residues may be present from the consumption of pepperoni which has preservatives.

Chapter 8, Module 8

1. Highly processed foods are missing from the food pyramid on page 133 of your book.

2. <u>Good carbs</u>: whole fruits and vegetables, rice, oats; <u>Bad carbs</u>: highly refined foods made from grain

3. avocado, walnut, flaxseed   4. Coconut oil, maple syrup, honey, butter, organic whole wheat bread

5. Individual responses   6. Energy, membrane   7. matter   8. Omega-3, omega-6

9. Individual responses, see page 136   10. See page 135, individual responses   11. Trans

12. See page 135. These foods are highly processed.   13. Crab, shrimp, salmon, clam

14. True   15. Individual responses   16. f, all the above   17. protein

18. A zinc finger is a protein high in zinc that is involved in cell division and repair, protein production, metabolism, and gene regulation.

19. See page 140, individual responses   20. Highly processed cereal and grain-based foods, nutrient poor meats (e.g. hot dogs, sausages, cold cuts) are what American children are eating when it comes to protein.

21. perform the work of cells and provide energy for making proteins   22. False

23. fatty liver disease   24. Non-alcoholic fatty liver disease (NAFLD)   25. True

26. obesity and all the associated disease conditions (e.g., type-2 diabetes, heart disease, cancer).

27. Individual responses.   28. Rinse fruit and vegetables under running water for 30 seconds

29. True   30. Individual responses

About Dr. Dufault

Dr. Renee J Dufault is a retired United States Public Health Service officer and an American research scientist who helped lay the foundation for the new field of study known as nutritional epigenetics. This field of study involves examining the diet and food supply to determine factors that may impact gene expression. Her first nutritional epigenetics study occurred when she was still working for the United States Food and Drug Administration (FDA) in 2006 after finding mercury residues in high fructose corn syrup samples collected by FDA law enforcement officers. According to the United States Department of Agriculture, Americans were each consuming up to 60 pounds per year high fructose corn syrup (HFCS) in 2005.

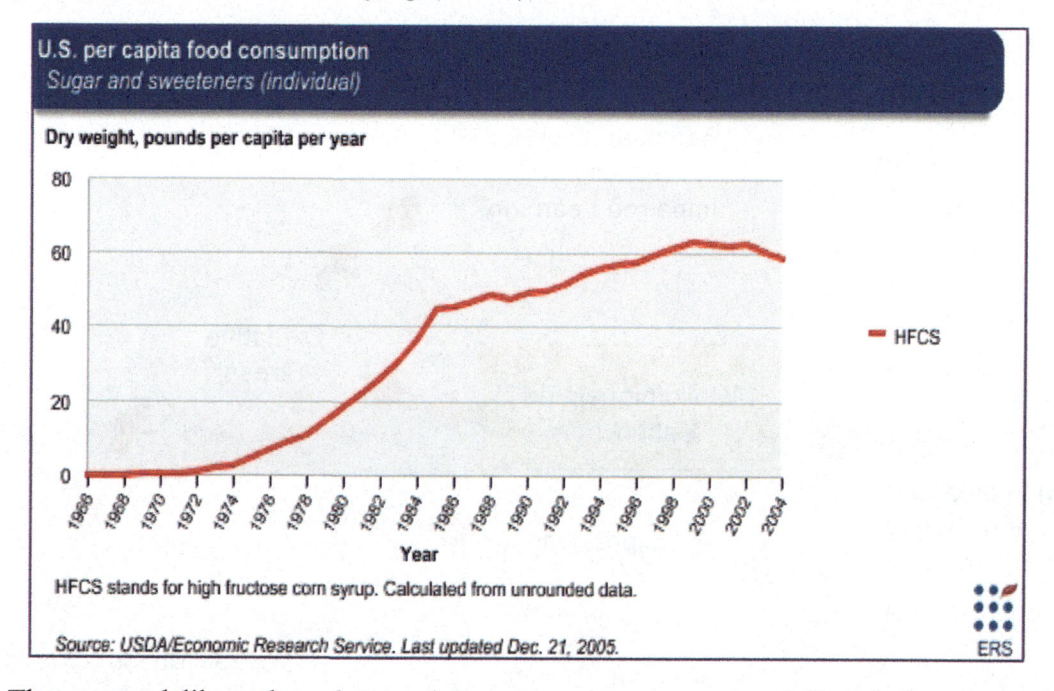

That seemed like a lot of potential mercury exposure especially when expectant mothers were reportedly consuming up to 60 pounds of corn syrup per year and corn syrup solids were commonly found in baby formulas. With her collaborator at the University of California at Davis, Dr. Isaac Pessah, she reported her findings and concerns to the FDA Center for Food Safety and Applied Nutrition (CFSAN). To her dismay, the FDA management commanded her to stop her investigation. Although she was no longer able to collect any more HFCS samples from the corn refiners, she still had some HFCS samples in storage at a different federal agency. These samples had their chain of custody intact. The collaborator at that agency agreed to store the samples until further notice.

Dr. Dufault remained concerned about the potential adverse impacts of the mercury exposures that were occurring in Americans from the consumption of HFCS. She became more concerned after conducting a review of the literature to determine how inorganic mercury exposures in the food supply may impact child development and learning. The focus of her study was on the effect of dietary/environmental mercury exposure via HFCS consumption on the MT gene. When the MT gene switches on, metallothionein protein is produced and the body uses this protein to detoxify and excrete heavy metals. During the literature review, Dr. Dufault discovered an article reporting the results of a study that determined the consumption of high fructose corn syrup leads to mineral imbalances in humans (e.g. zinc loss, copper gain). Dr. Dufault determined that the consumption of HFCS in great quantities could lead to zinc deficits that may impact the functioning of the MT gene, which is zinc dependent. Malfunction of the MT gene could lead to heavy metal accumulation and oxidative stress which may impair child learning. Dr. Dufault also determined in her literature review that with dietary selenium deficits, mercury exposures would be even more harmful because the glutathione anti-oxidant system would become ineffective. Dr. Dufault called her nutritional epigenetics model: The Mercury Toxicity Model. It was very simple. See figure below.

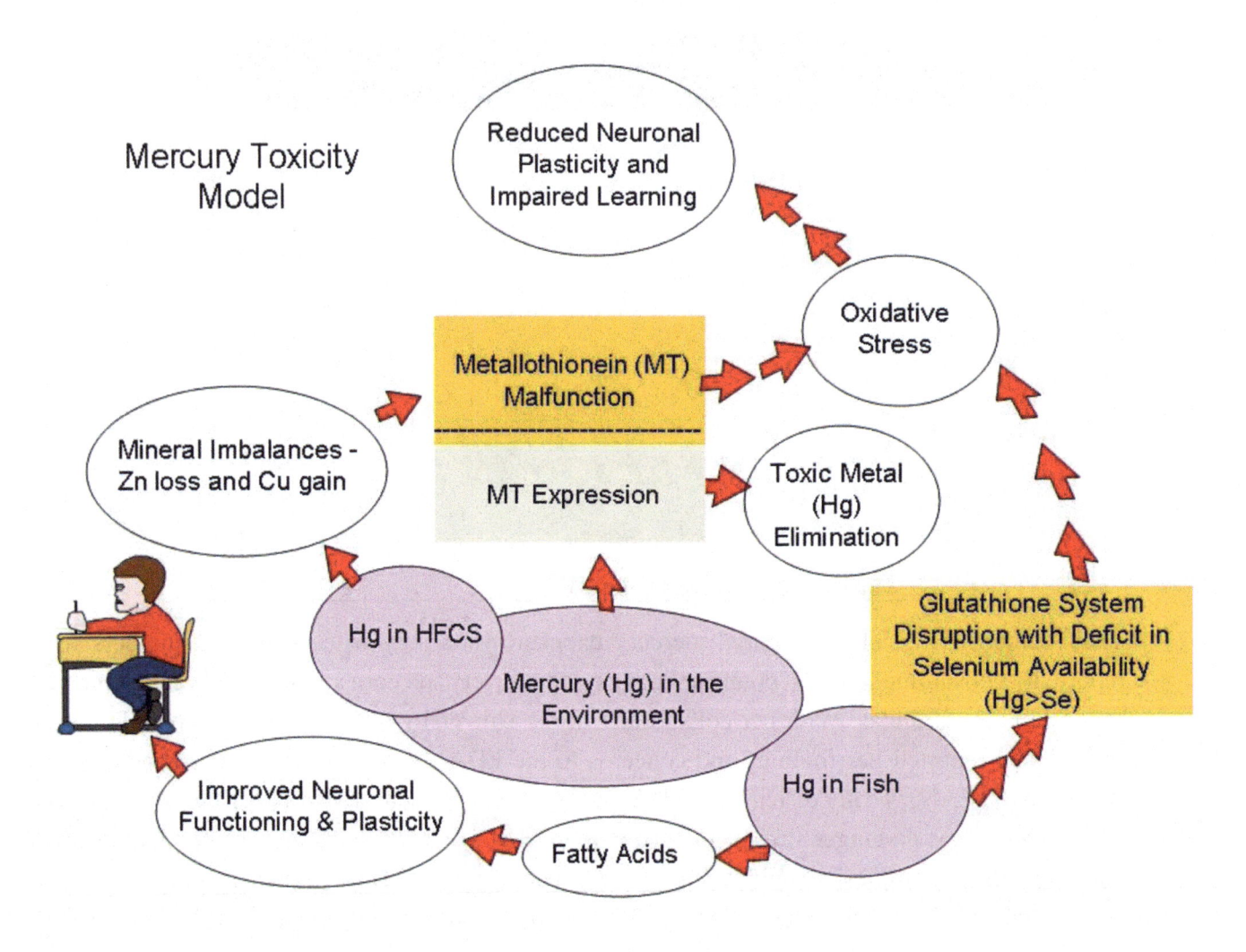

Unable to obtain additional HFCS samples for analysis, Dr. Dufault worked with collaborators outside of the government to write a report of her findings in a manuscript to be published in a peer reviewed medical journal. Unfortunately, to thwart the publication of these findings, the FDA upper management barred Dr. Dufault from using the laboratory data she obtained while working at FDA.

Specifically, Dr. Dufault had a written report from the National Institute of Standards and Technology (NIST) showing the mercury levels found in the HFCS samples. This was the only formal report she had, and she was barred from using it. The manuscript had to be set aside for the time being.

Dr. Dufault prepared to retire early from her career to continue the line of research. She was given permission to have the remaining HFCS samples in cold storage at another federal agency transferred by chain-of-custody to the University of Wisconsin for later analysis. Dr. Dufault retired from the FDA at the end of 2007 and continued her collaboration with researchers at the University of Wisconsin and other organizations. New analytical results became available and Dr. Dufault and her collaborators were finally able to publish the finding of mercury in HFCS in one manuscript and the literature review results with the Mercury Toxicity Model in another manuscript in 2009.

Since her retirement in 2007, Dr. Dufault has continued her line of research in the field of nutritional epigenetics. With her collaborators, she revised the original Mercury Toxicity Model as new data became available in the literature. In a second literature review, Dr. Dufault discovered a study conducted by US Department of Agriculture researchers who found consumption of HFCS leads to calcium losses in humans when dietary magnesium intake is low. Dr. Dufault identified a calcium dependent gene that is involved in autism and ADHD and suppressed by both dietary fructose and heavy metal exposures. Calcium deficits, dietary fructose, and mercury and lead exposures all suppress the PON1 gene. See Revised Mercury Toxicity Model below:

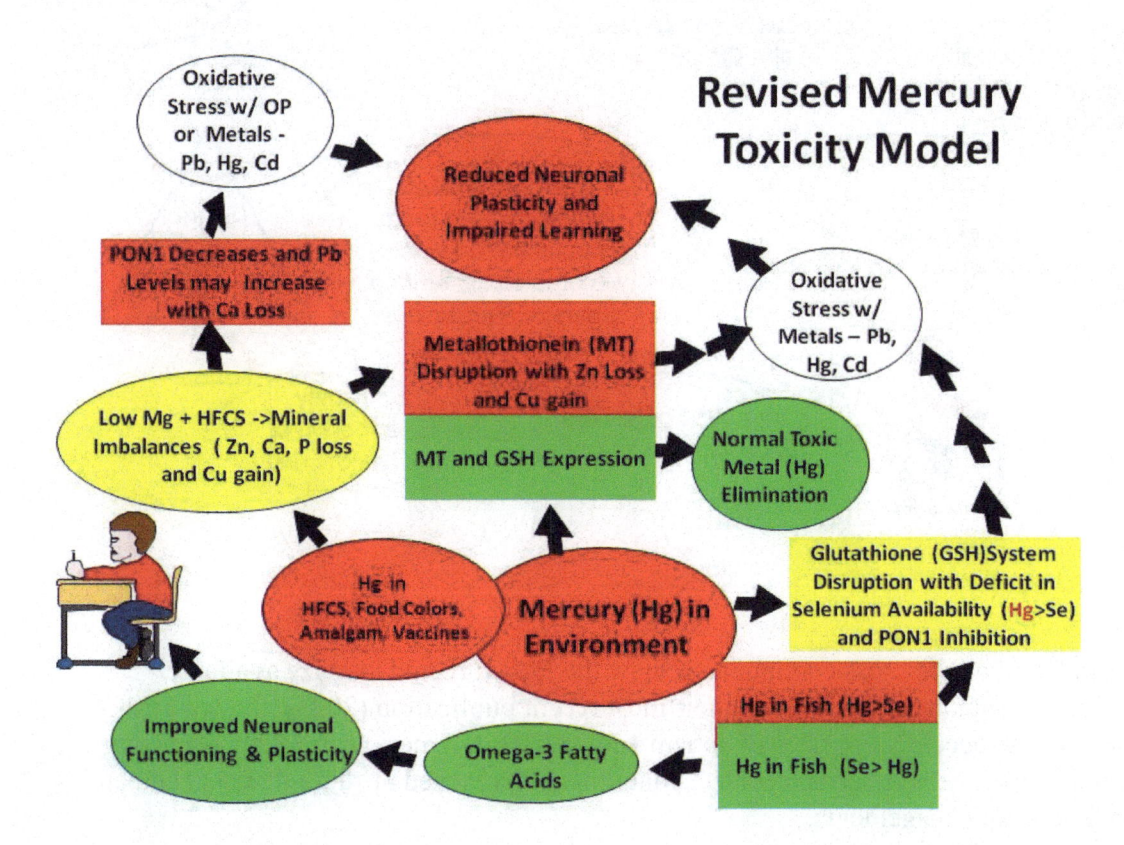

Suppression of the PON1 gene disables the body's ability to detoxify organophosphate pesticides. Children with autism and ADHD have lower PON1 gene activity and are thus susceptible to organophosphate pesticide poisoning which further impairs their learning and brain functioning.

Since Dr. Dufault began her line of research, numerous clinical trial data now show that children with autism and/or ADHD bioaccumulate dietary inorganic mercury and/or lead in their red blood cells. In 2021, Dr. Dufault and her collaborative research team published guidelines for physicians to connect inorganic mercury and lead measurements in blood to dietary sources of exposure in these disabled children. The guidelines also provide recommendations for dietary changes to reduce heavy metal exposures and reduce symptoms in children with autism and ADHD. The new nutritional epigenetics model is called Mercury and Lead Toxicity model for autism and ADHD and published in the *World Journal of Methodology*. See new nutritional epigenetics model below:

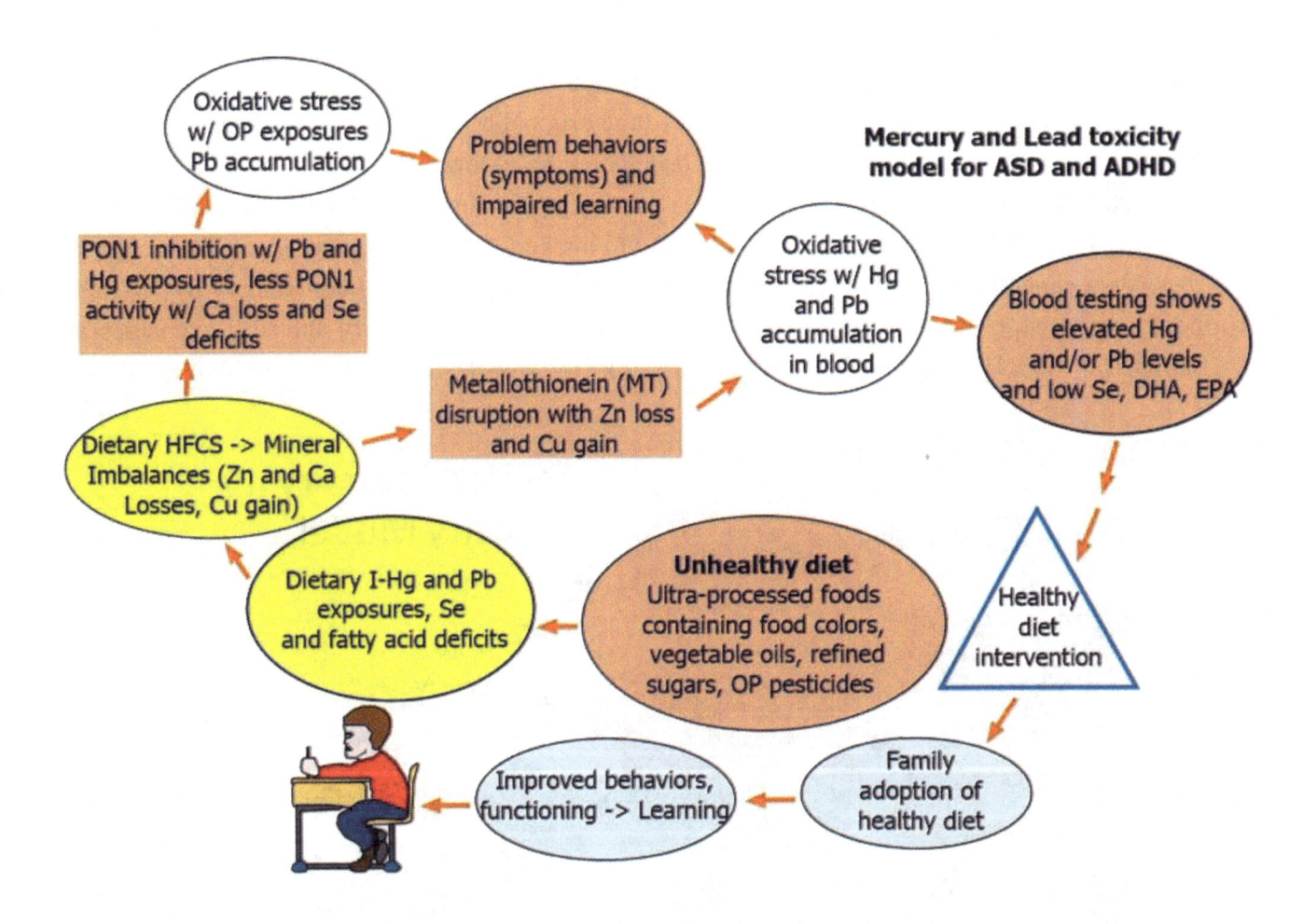

Mercury and Lead toxicity model for ASD and ADHD

- Oxidative stress w/ OP exposures Pb accumulation
- Problem behaviors (symptoms) and impaired learning
- Oxidative stress w/ Hg and Pb accumulation in blood
- Blood testing shows elevated Hg and/or Pb levels and low Se, DHA, EPA
- PON1 inhibition w/ Pb and Hg exposures, less PON1 activity w/ Ca loss and Se deficits
- Metallothionein (MT) disruption with Zn loss and Cu gain
- Dietary HFCS -> Mineral Imbalances (Zn and Ca Losses, Cu gain)
- Dietary I-Hg and Pb exposures, Se and fatty acid deficits
- Unhealthy diet: Ultra-processed foods containing food colors, vegetable oils, refined sugars, OP pesticides
- Healthy diet intervention
- Family adoption of healthy diet
- Improved behaviors, functioning -> Learning

Dr. Dufault and her collaborators continue to review the literature and analyze available prevalence data for autism and ADHD. In their most recent publication (2023), they publish evidence to show the accelerating rates of autism and ADHD in America are likely occurring via transgenerational epigenetic inheritance. Dr. Dufault may be reached at rdufault@atsu.edu and is available for speaking engagements.

References

1. Dufault et al. (2009). **Mercury from chlor-alkali plants: measured concentrations in food product sugar**. *Environmental Health*, 8:2. Mercury from chlor-alkali plants: measured concentrations in food product sugar - PubMed (nih.gov)

2. Dufault et al. (2009). **Mercury exposure, nutritional deficiencies and metabolic disruptions may affect learning in children.** *Behavioral and Brain Functions,* 5:44. Mercury exposure, nutritional deficiencies and metabolic disruptions may affect learning in children - PubMed (nih.gov)

3. Dufault et al. (2012). **A macroepigenetic to identify factors responsible for the autism epidemic in the United States**. *Clinical Epigenetics,* 4:6. A macroepigenetic approach to identify factors responsible for the autism epidemic in the United States - PubMed (nih.gov)

4. Dufault et al. (2015). **Blood inorganic mercury is directly associated with glucose levels in the human population and may be linked to processed food intake**. *Integrative Molecular Medicine*, 2(3):166-179. Blood inorganic mercury is directly associated with glucose levels in the human population and may be linked to processed food intake - PubMed (nih.gov)

5. Dufault R. and Gilbert S. (Oct. 23, 2017). **Why does autism impact boys more often than girls?** *Scientific American*. https://blogs.scientificamerican.com/observations/why-does-autism-impact-boys-more-often-than-girls/

6. Dufault R. (2017). **Unsafe at Any Meal: What the FDA Does Not Want You to Know About the Foods You Eat.** Square One Publishers: Garden City, NY.

7. Dufault et al. (2021). **Connecting inorganic mercury and lead measurements in blood to dietary sources of exposure that may impact child development**. *World Journal of Methodology*, 11(4):144-159. Connecting inorganic mercury and lead measurements in blood to dietary sources of exposure that may impact child development - PubMed (nih.gov)

8. Dufault et al. (2023). **Higher rates of autism and attention deficit/hyperactivity disorder in American children: Are food quality issues impacting epigenetic inheritance?** *World Journal of Clinical Pediatrics* 12(2): 25-37. Higher rates of autism and ADHD in American children: Are food quality issues impacting epigenetic inheritance?

SELECTED MEDIA LINKS

PubMed renee dufault - Search Results - PubMed (nih.gov)
Google Scholar [721 citations]
https://scholar.google.com/citations?user=EhXJgfgAAAAJ&hl=en
Wikipedia Page https://en.wikipedia.org/wiki/Renee_Dufault

CONTACT INFORMATION

Dr. Renee Dufault, E-mail: rdufault@atsu.edu

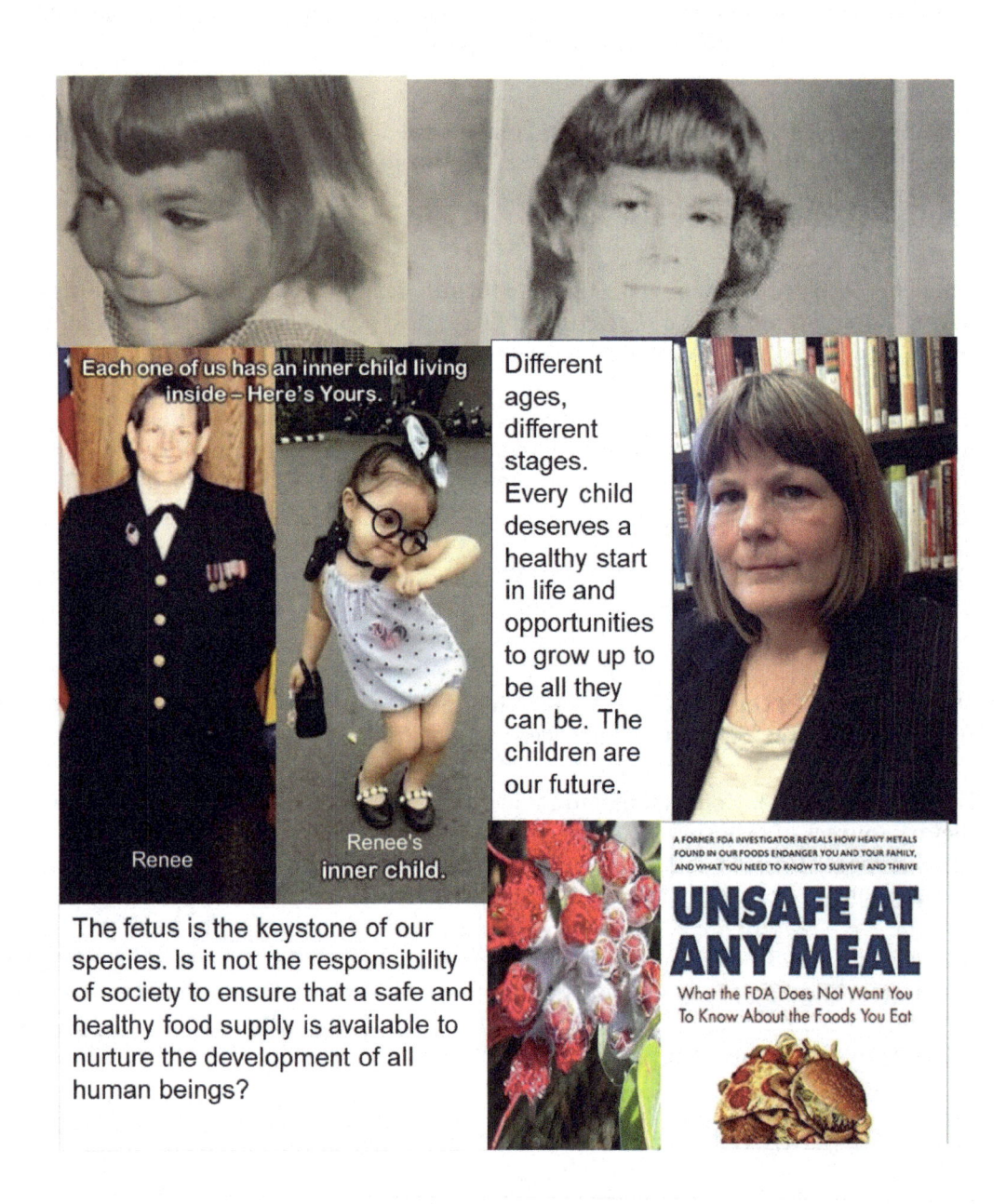

Made in the USA
Columbia, SC
02 May 2023